Advances in Applied Neurological Sciences 5

Editors
R. J. Joynt, Rochester, USA
A. Weindl, Munich, FRG

Drug-Induced Headache

Edited by
H.-C. Diener and M. Wilkinson

With 26 Figures and 74 Tables

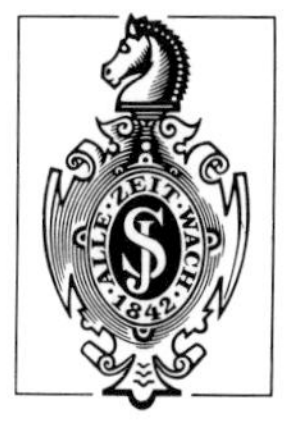

Springer-Verlag
Berlin Heidelberg New York
London Paris Tokyo

Hans-Christoph Diener, MD, Prof. of Neurology
Department of Neurology, University of Tübingen
Liebermeisterstr. 18–20, 7400 Tübingen, FRG

Marcia Wilkinson, MA, DM, FRCP
The City of London Migraine Clinic
22 Charterhouse Square
London EC1M 6DX, United Kingdom

ISBN 3-540-18762-6 Springer-Verlag Berlin Heidelberg New York
ISBN 0-387-18762-6 Springer-Verlag New York Berlin Heidelberg

Library of Congress Cataloging in Publication Data. Drug-induced headache. (Advances in applied neurological sciences; 5) Includes bibliographies and index. 1. Headache. 2. Drugs–Side effects. I. Diener, H.-C. (Hans-Christoph), 1951– . II. Wilkinson, Marcia. III. Series. [DNLM: 1. Drug Therapy–adverse effect. 2. Headache–chemically induced W1 AD436AH v. 5 / WL 342 D794] RB128.D78 1988 615′.7042 88-4479 ISBN 0-387-18762-6 (U.S.)

Typesetting, printing and bookbinding: Brühlsche Universitätsdruckerei, Giessen
2125/3130-543210

Contents

Pharmacological Aspects of Drug-Induced Headache

Treatment of Drug-Induced Headache

List of Contributors

You will find the addresses at the beginning of the respective contribution

Introduction

M. WILKINSON

Patients with frequent or daily headaches pose a very difficult problem for the physician who has to treat them, particularly as many patients think that there should be a medicine or medicines which give them instant relief. In the search for the compound which would meet this very natural desire, many drugs have been manufactured and the temptation for the physician is either to increase the dose of a drug which seems to be, at any rate, partially effective, or to add one or more drugs to those which the patient is already taking. Although there have been some references to the dangers of overdosage of drugs for migraine in the past, it was not until relatively recently that it was recognized that drugs given for the relief of headache, if taken injudiciously, may themselves cause headache. The first drugs to be implicated in this way were ergotamine and phenazone. In the case of ergotamine tartrate, the dangers of ergotism were well known as this was a disorder which had been known and written about for many years. In the treatment of headache, fully blown ergotism is rare and in recent years has usually been due to self-medication in doses much greater than those prescribed although there are a few recorded cases where toxic amounts have been given. The fact that patients could become habituated to ergot in what were then considered therapeutic doses was not fully recognized until the 1960s or 1970s, and, until the early 1970s, at least one reputable international pharmaceutical company was suggesting that doses of up to 24 mg of ergotamine tartrate a week were acceptable. This contrasts with the present view that ergotamine should only be taken once or twice a week and that the maximum dose should probably not exceed 6 mg per week.

Patients taking regular doses of ergotamine tartrate appear to become habituated to the drug. "Habituation" can be defined as the constant use of a drug, deprivation of which causes symptoms of distress which is accompanied by an irresistible impulse to take the drug. In the case of ergotamine tartrate, headache, or the fear of a headache developing, is the trigger for taking more because once the patient has become habituated to it, the headaches are only relieved by further doses.

Phenazone is another drug which, taken regularly, may cause headache when taken for the relief of headache. This aspect of phenazone overdose was slow to be recognized because of the other more serious aspects of toxicity such as nephropathy. Once the dangers of this drug were realized, its use was severely restricted.

The City of London Migraine Clinic, 22 Charterhouse Square, London, ECIM 6DX, United Kingdom

Drug-Induced Headache
Ed. by H.-C. Diener and M. Wilkinson
© Springer-Verlag Berlin Heidelberg 1988

Simple analgesics such as aspirin and paracetamol (acetaminophen) have only recently been recognized as potential causes of daily headache, but in the last 10 years the constant use of analgesics has been shown to be one of the causes of chronic headaches.

This book has been written by acknowledged experts on chronic drug abuse as the cause of headache and deals with many aspects of the problem. All authors agree that where possible the offending drug should be stopped, preferably abruptly, and, if the patient cannot manage this on his own, hospitalization may be necessary. The immediate results are good, but, as in other types of dependency, there is a high relapse rate and unless the patient is given continued support the problem may reoccur.

During the Second International Workshop on Drug-Related Headache at the University of Tuebingen in 1986, the participating experts agreed on the following definition for drug-related headache:

1. More than 20 headache days per month
2. Daily headache duration exceeding 10 h
3. Intake of analgesic or migraine drugs on more than 20 days per month
4. Regular intake of analgesics and/or ergotamine preparations in combination with barbiturates, codeine, caffeine, antihistaminics or tranquillizers
5. Increase in the severity and frequency of headaches after discontinuation of drug intake (rebound headache)
6. The nature of the underlying headache, e.g. migraine, tension headache, cluster headache, post-traumatic headache or cervicogenic headache, is not related to the syndrome.

Clinical Aspects of Drug-Induced Headache

Daily Chronic Headache – Tension Headaches, Migraine, and Combined Headaches: The Transformation Concept

J. R. Saper

This short introduction will emphasize the approach to chronic recurring daily or almost daily headache and it will consider the phenomenon of "migraine transformation" in which episodic and typical primary headache conditions appear to be transformed into chronic daily headache patterns. In 1962, the Ad Hoc Committee on Classification of Headache offered what was to become the standard classification for head pain disorders for the next 20 years. This report was based upon the premise of a clear distinction between migraine and tension headache (TH) and emphasized system-specific etiologies: vasculature in migraine, musculature in tension headache. But, despite its many citations and its traditional acceptance by researchers and clinicians alike, many authorities have been unable to reconcile the myriad of events and phenomena of migraine, TH, and cluster headache with the basic foundations of this classification. During the past few years, the emphasis on peripheral phenomena (blood vessels and muscles) and separateness between migraine and TH disorders has been challenged, and with it has come a change views on the treatment of these disorders.

Clinicians are now citing data that they believe support the view that migraine and TH are physiologically related entities, reflecting a varied symptomatic expression of central (brain) disturbances (transmitter or receptor function) within the upper brainstem, limbic and/or hypothalamic regions (Saper 1986). Moreover, many authorities of headache are now suggesting that tension may be less a disorder of muscle than a chronic disturbance of neural function with muscle factors playing a secondary role.

This "central hypothesis" gains its support from several observations. Among these are current understanding of brain mechanisms including the neurochemical and physiological events which are purported to occur during headache; the symptom overlap between migraine and TH; the fact that a considerable number of patients experience both migraine and TH; the general acknowledgement that the clinical phenomena, including pain, cannot be satisfactorily or entirely explained by disturbances of vascular or muscular structures; vascular flow studies which challenge traditional views linking preheadache and headache symptoms of migraine with specific changes in blood flow (Lauritzen and Olesen 1984); and therapeutic considerations which raise doubt as to the presumed mechanism of well-known therapeutic agents (Peatfield et al. 1986).

On this last point, drugs initially recognized to be useful for migraine or muscle contraction headache (e.g., anti-depressants) may be of value in both disorders. Moreover, a large number of agents found useful in the treatment of TH, migraine, or both conditions do not demonstrate a consistent system (vascular or

Michigan Headache and Neurological Institute, 3120 Professional Drive, Ann Arbor, MI 48104, USA

Drug-Induced Headache
Ed. by H.-C. Diener and M. Wilkinson
© Springer-Verlag Berlin Heidelberg 1988

muscular) specificity sufficient to explain their effectiveness. In fact, the wide-ranging pharmacological actions of drugs like beta-blocking agents, which are found useful in chronic headache disorders, appear to share influence on the central brain mechanisms more than a specific vascular or muscular effect.

The perspectives on chronic headache are changing, and the villains of the past 100 years (blood vessels and muscles) are now coming to be seen as possible victims, affected by chronic, intermittent, or continuous disturbances of central phenomena. Currently, the International Association for the Study of Headache is undertaking the first major attempt to reclassify headaches since the Ad Hoc Committee Report of 1962. Ironically, controversy and disagreement already exist as to terminology and mechanism.

"Migraine" was defined by the Ad Hoc Committee as:

Migraine is a familial disorder characterized by recurrent attacks of headache widely variable in intensity, frequency, and duration. Attacks are commonly unilateral and are usually associated with anorexia, nausea, and vomiting. In some cases, they are preceded by, or associated with, neurological and mood disturbances. All the above characteristics are not necessarily present in each attack or in each patient.

"Tension headache" was defined by the Ad Hoc Committee as:

Ache or sensation of tightness, pressure, or constriction, widely varied in intensity, frequency, and duration; longlasting, and commonly suboccipital, associated with sustained contraction of skeletal muscles – usually as part of the individual's reaction to life stress.

"Combined headaches" (vascular and muscle contraction) were defined as follows:

Combinations of vascular headache of the migraine type and muscle contraction headache commonly coexist in an attack.

Historically, physicians have used the term "tension headache" to characterize a daily or almost daily chronic headache disorder without vascular-type features and which is likely but not necessarily associated with provocation by stress or emotional factors. Migraine and muscle contraction headaches were considered distinct entities. In the German-speaking countries, the term "vasomotor headache" was used instead of "tension headache."

So imprecise are the criteria for TH, and so casually has the diagnosis been applied, that to many the diagnosis is but a "waste-basket" entity. The diagnosis has been rendered to any headache disorder which is ostensibly not vascular (migraine, cluster) nor associated with identifiable structural disease and which occurs when elements of stress, anxiety, or depression are evident.

The challenge to traditional views actually began with Dalessio's early observations regarding the central actions of drugs used in migraine (Dalessio et al. 1961; Dalessio 1980). Raskin and Appenzeller (1980), described a "clinical continuum" they believed to be primary to the basic migraine/TH disposition. Mathew (1982) and Dichgangs et al. (1984) described the transformation of intermittent migraine to "daily migraine." Saper (1983) and Saper et al. (1983) expanded this concept further, demonstrating a pattern of transformation that involved large numbers (515) of daily chronic headache patients. All patients had begun their headache course with intermittent typical migraine, but by 8–10 years following the onset, individuals were experiencing daily chronic headache, indistinguishable from the historical description of TH. Other features of this transformation included a high incidence of depression, sleep disturbance, and analgesic overusage. Family histories of these patients showed that over 90% of females and 84% of males had a close family relative with headache and a higher than expected incidence of substance abuse, alcoholism, and depression. Daily analgesic use was present in 77% of patients, and 26% demonstrated a neuroendocrine disturbance as reflected by abnormal cortisol suppression via the dexamethasone suppression test.

Several European studies have similarly emphasized a centrally determined transformational process. They define "common migraine" as an "evolutive disease" characterized by progressive increase in the number of attacks, a gradual reduction of headache-free periods, and eventually reaching the state of continuous migraine with interparoxysmal headache (MIH) (Nappi and Savoldi 1985; Micieli et al. this volume). The interparoxysmal headache is acute migraine superimposed upon daily chronic background.

It is likely that common migraine, continuous MIH vasomotor headache as defined by the Europeans, and the transformational syndromes as intimated by Raskin and Appenzeller and later specifically reported by Mathew et al. (1982) and detailed by this author (Saper 1983) are the same phenomena.

The basic etiology of drug-induced headache is still hypothetical. Central biochemical dysnociception, due to disturbances of the monoamine system and/or endorphin disturbances involving hypothalamic and brainstem mechanisms and hypothalamic chronobiologic control as well as changes in the responsiveness of cranial vessels to neurotransmitters could be possible mechanisms.

References

Ad Hoc Committee (1962) Classification of headache. JAMA 179:717–718

Dalessio DJ (1980) Wolff's headache and other pain (4th edn). Oxford University Press, New York

Dalessio DJ, Camp WA, Goodell H, Wolff HG (1961) Studies on headache. The mode of action of UML-491 in its relevance to the nature of vascular headache of the migraine type. Arch Neurol 4:235–240

Dichgans J, Diener HC, Gerber WD, Verspohl EJ, Kukiolka H, Kluck M (1984) Analgetikainduzierter Dauerkopfschmerz. Dtsch Med Wochenschr 109:369–373

Lauritzen M, Olesen J (1984) Regional cerebral blood flow during migraine attacks by Xenon-133 inhalation and emission tomography. Brain 107:447–461

Mathew NT, Stubits SE, Nigam M (1982) Transformation of migraine into daily headache: analysis of factors. Headache 22:66–68

Nappi G, Savoldi F (1985) Headache. Diagnostic system and taxonomic criteria. Libbey, London

Peatfield RC, Fozzard JR, Clifford Rose F (1986) Drug treatment of migraine. In: Clifford Rose F (ed) Handbook of clinical neurology, vol 4 (48): Headache. Elsevier, Amsterdam, pp 173–216

Raskin NH, Appenzeller O (1980) Headache. Saunders Philadelphia

Saper JR (1983) Headache disorders: current concepts and treatment strategies. Wright PSG, Littleton Massachusetts

Saper JR (1986) Changing perspectives on chronic headache. Clin J Pain 2:19–28

Saper JR, Johnson T, van Meter M (1983) "Mixed headache": a chronic headache complex: a study of 500 patients. Headache 23:143

Clinical Manifestations of Excessive Use of Analgesic Medication

J. Dichgans and H.-C. Diener

Physicians experienced in the treatment of migraine and other forms of headache are nowadays well aware that the daily intake of antipyretic or anti-inflammatory analgesics or combinations with ergotamine, sedatives, or hypnotics may result in chronic daily headache. Conversely, if a patient complains of daily headache and takes "pain killers" daily, this headache is most likely to be caused and sustained by the medication and will vanish with abstinence. Chronic headache was originally attributed to the excessive use of ergotamine preparations (Lippman 1955; Horton and Peters 1963; Lucas and Falkowski 1973; Rowsell et al. 1973; Wainscott et al. 1974; Andersson 1975; Dige-Petersen et al. 1977; Hokkanen et al. 1978; Ala-Hurula et al. 1982; Pradalier et al. 1984) and was therefore named "ergotamine headache." A number of subsequent reports from different countries in Western Europe and the United States, however, indicated that analgesics may induce chronic headache as well (Wörz et al. 1975; Medina and Diamond 1977; Tfelt-Hansen and Krabbe 1981; Kudrow 1982; Isler 1982; Wörz 1983; Dichgans et al. 1984; Henry et al. 1985; Rapaport et al. 1985). We, therefore, propose to add to the original terms "ergotamine headache" and "analgesic headache" a new entity and to include both under the term "drug-induced headache."

Epidemiology of Analgesic Intake

Exact numbers giving the frequency of analgesic intake and abuse are not available. "Analgesic abuse" in this respect is defined as the regular daily intake of analgesics, resulting in tolerance with unchanged symptoms (e.g., headache) or increasing dosages and withdrawal symptoms after the discontinuation of daily medication. An estimate of the average intake of pain killers can be obtained by looking at the sales of analgesics and migraine drugs in the Federal Republic of Germany. In 1982 113 142 200 packs of analgesics and 8 903 600 packs of migraine drugs were sold (Langbein et al. 1983). Even if we assume that the smallest packages were bought, this would mean that every single inhabitant consumed 37 tablets within 1 year. If one assumes that only one in ten consumed analgesics, this means that every person took on average one tablet per day. The sales of analgesic combinations containing between 40 and 250 tablets per pack exceeded 4.5 million in 1983 (Mihatsch et al. 1986).

Department of Neurology, University of Tübingen, Liebermeisterstr. 18–20, 7400 Tübingen 1, Federal Republic of Germany

Drug-Induced Headache
Ed. by H.-C. Diener and M. Wilkinson
© Springer-Verlag Berlin Heidelberg 1988

There are 256 brands of analgesics sold in the Federal Republic of Germany. Only 43 contain a single drug (27 salicylic acid = aspirin, 13 acetaminophen = paracetamol, and three metamizole). All other brands are combinations, 12 of which contain barbiturates, and 33 codeine. Eight of 46 brands sold for migraine therapy contain one substance only including barbiturates, lisuride, methysergide, pizotifen, ergotamine, and clonidine. All other drugs are combinations and often contain barbiturates and codeine. In some cases, up to nine (!) single substances are found in one tablet.

Interviews of a representative sample of the Swiss population revealed that 4.4% of men and 6.8% of women took analgesics at least once a week (Gutzwiller and Zemp 1986). A total of 2.3% admitted to taking these drugs every day. Inpatient records from several departments of psychiatry in Switzerland between 1974 and 1977 showed that dependency on analgesics was more frequent than dependency on tranquilizers, hypnotics, and stimulating drugs (Kielholz and Ladewig 1981). A prevalence study performed in 1979 in Austria included 3182 persons aged between 25 and 80 years. All subjects were asked about regular or frequent intake of drugs. Between 5% and 9% of men and 13%–21% of all women between 25 and 60 years admitted the frequent intake of headache medication. The amount taken depended on the age and increased with age. The number of people taking analgesics outnumbered those taking hypnotics, tranquilizers, and laxatives (Porpaczy 1986). Calculations from the number of tablets sold indicate that possibly 1% of the population in the Federal Republic of Germany take up to ten pain killers every day (Schwarz et al. 1985).

Analgesic Syndrome

In addition to chronic headache there may be other symptoms suggesting the analgesic syndrome (Mihatsch 1986). These depend on the duration and amount of drugs consumed. They are:

- Chronic headache
- Drug dependency
- Nephropathy
- Gastrointestinal disorders
- Cardiovascular disorders (including ergotism)
- Hematological disorders
- Dry hair and gray skin

From a historical point of view, it is interesting to observe the divergent approach to this problem by neurologists on the one side and nephrologists on the other. Neurologists were usually confronted with the symptom of chronic headache whereas physicians practicing internal medicine saw patients after more than 20 years of analgesic abuse. By this time, chronic renal failure had developed and hemodialysis or renal transplantation had to be considered. Nowadays, the diagnosis and cure of analgesic abuse and analgesic nephropathy is the responsibility of every physician who treats headache patients.

Prevalence in Women

Analgesic abuse is more frequent in women than in men. This can be shown for both chronic headache (see Table 2, Diener et al., this volume) and analgesic nephropathy (Stewart 1978; Dubach 1986). In our first study of 52 patients (Dichgans et al. 1984), 12 times as many women had analgesic headache. In a further study of 179 patients (unpublished), five times as many women were diagnosed as suffering from analgesic headache. Examination of the patient may give hints of the diagnosis. Most of the women look much older than they are, have gray skin and sparse dry hair. Many patients complain about asthenia, loss of weight, cold feet, sleep disturbances, and depression.

Chronic Headache

Drug-induced headache persists typically throughout the entire day. It is already present in the early morning when patients awake, and the pain is frequently localized in the neck (Andersson 1975). The headache differs in intensity and in most cases is described as being diffuse and dull in character with either frontal or occipital accentuation (Kudrow 1982). In some patients, it may spread along both parietal bones (Lippman 1955). Patients are never headache free and may experience in addition migraine attacks with hemicrania, nausea, vomiting, and photophobia. All patients found that the intensity of the headache increased whenever they tried to stop medication (rebound headache; Lucas and Falkowski 1973).

The mechanism which leads to chronic headache with analgesics is unclear. Ergot alkaloids lead to a long-lasting vasoconstriction (see Tfelt-Hansen, this volume). The decrease in plasma levels during the night might be one factor explaining why patients wake up in the morning with headache and why they tend to take medication late in the evening so as to avoid this. Changes in the prostaglandin metabolism may be responsible for chronic headache as salicylic acid as well as nonsteroidal anti-inflammatory drugs may cause headache. This has been insufficiently investigated. The combination of drugs, in particular combinations of barbiturates with stimulating ingredients, seems to promote drug abuse and the subsequent chronification of headache (Isler 1982; Dichgans et al. 1984). Whether these substances play a part in the causation of daily headache is not entirely clear. Monosubstances should be used whenever possible.

Drug Dependency

The psychotropic side effects of analgesic or migraine drugs, such as sedation or mild euphoria, and their stimulating action may lead to drug dependency. Barbiturates, codeine, and caffeine are the most likely substances to have this effect.

Caffeine increases vigilance, relieves fatigue, improves performance and mood. The typical symptoms of caffeine withdrawal, such as irritability, nervousness, restlessness, and especially "caffeine withdrawal headache" (Greden et al. 1980; Abbott 1986) which may last for several days, encourage the patients to continue their abuse. Despite the fact that caffeine may enhance the analgesic action of salicylic acid and acetaminophen (Laska et al. 1984), it should be removed from analgesics.

There are only rare reports on physical dependence on codeine. As far as we know, there are no studies which have investigated the effects of codeine intake over periods as long as 10 years. Many of our patients have taken it for this length of time. It should be remembered that up to 10% of codeine is metabolized to morphine (Meadows 1984).

Ergotamine may certainly lead to physical dependency (Saper and Jones 1986). Many patients who feel a migraine attack coming on may take ergotamine as prophylactic treatment. Professional women are particularly likely to do this (e.g., teachers; Dichgans et al. 1984). The drugs may improve performance, at least subjectively, and the patient, without being aware of it, progressively changes the goal of self-medication. Finally, the rebound headache confirms the patient's attitude that he is better with than without the drugs.

Nephropathy

In 1950, Spühler and Zollinger realized for the first time the causal relationship between the ingestion of large quantities of analgesic drugs (phenacetin) and nephropathy. Morphologically, analgesic nephropathy is characterized by papillary necrosis and tubulointerstitial inflammation. The prevalence of phenacetin abusers at autopsy as revealed by the typical nephropathy was between 1.8% and 3.2% in a population study in Switzerland (Mihatsch et al. 1980a, b).

A significant percentage of patients requiring hemodialysis or renal transplantation are abusers of analgesics. The combined report on regular dialysis and transplantation in Europe estimated that between 0.9% and 32.5% of all patients with chronic renal failure had toxic nephropathy (Gutzwiller and Zemp 1986). Phenacetin and combinations of other analgesics are most likely to cause this disease. A 9-year prospective follow-up study in 623 women frequently taking analgesics containing phenacetin compared with 622 women without regular analgesic intake showed significantly increased serum creatinin levels, increased mortality, and increased numbers of urinary tract disorders in the former group (Dubach et al. 1978, 1983).

The correlation between phenacetin intake and nephropathy is proved by the decreasing frequency of toxic nephropathy after the ban of phenacetin in Denmark and Sweden in 1961 (from 10% in 1970 to 2% in 1980). In Canada, phenacetin was removed from over-the-counter medication in 1970. In 1972, the Canadian government ordered the removal of phenacetin from all mixtures and banned combinations of salicylic acid and acetaminophen. Analgesic nephropathy decreased by more than 50% during the next 9 years (Korcak 1980). In the Federal Republic of Germany, phenacetin was removed from analgesics in 1985 and 1986.

At least 2 kg phenacetin must be taken over a period to cause nephropathy. In addition, analgesic abusers have a five- to ten-fold higher risk of suffering from malignant tumors of the kidneys and the urinary collecting system (Mihatsch and Knüsli 1982; Mihatsch et al. 1982b) than the population as a whole. The incidence of urinary tract tumors was 8.6% at autopsy of phenacetin abusers and 1.7% in control subjects. 52% of the malignant tumors were localized in the bladder, 42% in the renal pelvis, and 6% in the ureter. Similar results were obtained in a case-control study by Piper et al. (1985). The average time interval from the beginning of phenacetin abuse to the occurrence of the tumor is 20–30 years, the cumulative drug intake 6–18 kg. Salicylic acid and acetaminophen seem to be less dangerous in this respect (Stewart 1978), but the possible consequences of combinations of these analgesics on kidney function are still unknown. There is new evidence that nonsteroidal anti-inflammatory drugs may cause renal failure (Adams et al. 1986). These drugs can also induce chronic headache.

Hematological Disorders

Anemia is seen in patients with regular intake of salicylic acid and in most cases it is due to chronic gastrointestinal hemorrhage. Anemia can also be caused by concomitant nephropathy. Aplastic anemia and agranulocytosis are very rarely reported after intake of pyrazolone derivates and salicylic acid, and never after acetaminophen. Phenylbutazone, acetaminophen, and salicylic acid may lead to thrombocytopenia.

Gastrointestinal Disorders

Salicylic acid (=aspirin) may cause erosive gastritis and, especially when taken together with alcohol, may lead to peptic ulcers and gastrointestinal hemorrhages. These side effects are well known from the prophylactic use of salicylic acid in cerebrovascular disease. Acetaminophen (=paracetamol) and metamizole do not affect the ventricular mucosa. Paracetamol taken in high dosages may cause liver disease (Meadows 1984). An autopsy study in Switzerland performed on 160 phenacetin abusers and 160 controls revealed a significantly higher number of gastric ulcers in the first group (Mihatsch et al. 1982a). Most of the phenacetin abusers, however, used mixed drugs.

Cardiovascular Disorders

A prospective study performed in Switzerland between 1968 and 1979 in patients with analgesic abuse showed that in addition to increased mortality due to kidney failure there was a significant increase in deaths from cardiovascular disorders (Dubach et al. 1983). At autopsy, it was found that cardiovascular disease was four times as frequent in phenacetin abusers as in controls (Mihatsch et al. 1983). The exact mechanism of this phenomenon is not yet fully understood. Some relevant changes are, however, known in this group of patients: they include increased occurrence of hypertension and increases in cholesterol levels.

Another risk factor might be the regular intake of ergotamine. There are even some reports summarized by Benedict and Robertson (1979) indicating that angina pectoris and sudden death can occur following ergotamine therapy for migraine. Ergotamine may cause acrocyanosis, intermittent claudication, and muscle cramps (Horton and Peters 1963; Saper and Jones 1986). Concerning the intensity and duration of ergotamine headache, there is, however, a low correlation between ergotamine headache, the serum levels of ergotamine measured, and the occurrence of clinical ergotism in single subjects (Ala-Hurula et al. 1982). A close analysis of 44 patients with ergotamine headache showed that 36% of the patients complained of cold feet and 13% had intermittent claudication (Andersson 1975). Measuring foot systolic blood pressure in patients who had taken ergotamine for more than 2 years revealed subclinical ergotism in most of them (Dige-Petersen et al. 1977).

Conclusions

In conclusion, the dangerous consequences of regular intake of analgesic combinations and migraine drugs should result in the following demands:

1. The number of analgesic tablets in any one package should be reduced to ten
2. Mixtures containing analgesics and barbiturates, tranquilizers, or other sedatives should be banned
3. The advertisement of headache and antimigraine drugs should be prohibited
4. All analgesic combinations should be banned

Summary

Regular intake of antipyretic or anti-inflammatory analgesics may cause a well-delineated syndrome of abuse, the analgesic syndrome. This is particularly likely to occur if ergotamine, sedatives, or hypnotics are also taken. The main symptoms are chronic daily headache and signs of drug dependency. The analgesic syndrome is more common in women. In the later stages, the abuse may lead to nephropathy, gastrointestinal, cardiovascular, and hematological disorders.

References

Abbott PJ (1986) Caffeine: a toxicological overview. Med J Aust 145:518–521

Adams DH, Howie AJ, Michael J, McConkey B, Bacon PA, Adu D (1986) Non-steroidal anti-inflammatory drugs and renal failure. Lancet i:57–59

Ala-Hurula V, Myllylä V, Hokkanen E (1982) Ergotamine abuse: results of ergotamine discontinuation with special reference to the plasma concentrations. Cephalalgia 2:189–195

Andersson PG (1975) Ergotamine headache. Headache 15:118–121

Benedict CR, Robertson D (1979) Angina pectoris and sudden death in the absence of atherosclerosis following ergotamine therapy for migraine. Am J Med 67:177–178

Dichgans J, Diener HC, Gerber WD, Verspohl EJ, Kukiolka H, Kluck M (1984) Analgetika-induzierter Dauerkopfschmerz. Dtsch Med Wochenschr 109:369–373

Dige-Petersen H, Lassen NA, Noer J, Toennesen KH, Olesen J (1977) Subclinical ergotism. Lancet II:65–66

Dubach UC (1986) Epidemiologische Untersuchungen zur Analgetikanephropathie. In: Mihatsch MJ (ed) Das Analgetikasyndrom. Thieme, Stuttgart, pp 47–53

Dubach UC, Rosner PS, Baumeler HR, Müller A, Peyer A, Ehrensperger T, Ettlin C (1978) Epidemiological study in Switzerland. Kidney Int 13:41–49

Dubach UC, Rosner B, Pfister E (1983) Epidemiologic study of abuse of analgesics containing phenacetin. Renal morbidity and mortality (1968–1979). N Engl J Med 308:357–362

Greden J, Victor B, Fontaine B, Lubetsky M (1980) Caffeine withdrawal: a clinical profile. Psychosomatics 21:411–418

Gutzwiller F, Zemp E (1986) Der Analgetikakonsum in der Bevölkerung und sozioökonomische Aspekte des Analgetikaabusus. In: Mihatsch MJ (ed) Das Analgetikasyndrom. Thieme, Stuttgart, pp 19–25

Henry P, Dartigues JF, Benetier MP, Lucas J, Duplan B, Jogeix M, Orgogozo JM (1985) Ergotamine- and analgesic-induced headaches. In: Rose FC (ed) Migraine. Proceedings 5th International Migraine Symposion London 1984. Karger, Basel, pp 197–205

Hokkanen E, Waltimo O, Kallaurata T (1978) Toxic effects of ergotamine used for migraine. Headache 18:95–98

Horton BT, Peters GA (1963) Clinical manifestations of excessive use of ergotamine preparations and management of withdrawal effect: report of 52 cases. Headache 3:214–226

Isler H (1982) Migraine treatment as a cause of chronic migraine. In: Rose FC (ed) Advances in migraine research and therapy. Raven, New York, pp 159–164

Kielholz P, Ladewig D (1981) Probleme des Medikamentenmißbrauches. Schweiz Ärzte Ztg 62:2866–2869

Korcak M (1981) Analgesic nephropathy dips in Canada after mixture ban. J Am Med Assoc 246:2008

Kudrow L (1982) Paradoxical effects of frequent analgesic use. In: Critchley M, Friedman AP, Gorini S, Sicuteri F (eds) Advances in Neurology, vol 33. Raven, New York, pp 335–341

Langbein K, Martin HP, Sichrovsky P, Weiss H (1983) Bittere Pillen; Nutzen und Risiken der Arzneimittel. Kiepenheuer und Witsch, Köln

Laska EM, Sunshine A, Mueller F, Elvers WB, Siegel C, Rubin A (1984) Caffeine as an analgesic adjuvant. JAMA 251:1711–1718

Lippman CW (1955) Characteristic headache resulting from prolonged use of ergot derivates. J Nerv Ment Dis 121:270–273

Lucas RN, Falkowski W (1973) Ergotamine and methysergide abuse in patients with migraine. Br J Psychiatry 122:199–203

Meadows BJ (1984) Codeine combinations in clinical practice. Curr Ther Res 35:501–510

Medina J, Diamond S (1977) Drug dependency in patients with chronic headaches. Headache 17:12–14

Mihatsch MJ (1986) Das Analgetikasyndrom. Thieme, Stuttgart

Mihatsch MJ, Knüsli C (1982) Phenacetin abuse and malignant tumors. Klin Wochenschr 60:1339–1349

Mihatsch MJ, Hofer HO, Gutzwiller F, Brunner FP, Zollinger HU (1980a) Phenacetinabusus I. Häufigkeit, Pro-Kopf-Verbrauch und Folgekosten. Schweiz Med Wochenschr 110:108–115

Mihatsch MJ, Schmidlin P, Brunner FP, Hofer HO, Six P, Zollinger HU (1980 b) Phenacetinabusus II. Die chronisch renale Niereninsuffizienz im Basler Autopsiegut. Schweiz Med Wochenschr 110:116–124

Mihatsch MJ, Kernen R, Zollinger HU (1982 a) Phenacetinabusus VI: eine Autopsiestatistik unter besonderer Berücksichtigung extrarenaler Befunde. Schweiz Med Wochenschr 112:1383–1388

Mihatsch MJ, Brunner FP, Korteweg E, Rist M, Dalguen P, Thiel G (1982 b) Phenacetinabusus VII: Harnwegtumoren bei Dialysepatienten und Nierentransplantatträgern. Schweiz Med Wochenschr 112:1468–1472

Mihatsch MJ, Staehlin HB, Musfeld D, Perret E, Oberholzer M (1983) Phenacetin-Abusus: Kardiovaskuläre Risikofaktoren. Nieren- und Hochdruckkrankheiten 12:83–92

Mihatsch MJ, Molzahn M, Ritz E (1986) Analgetika-Abusus – ist das Phenacetinverbot ausreichend? Dtsch Med Wochenschr 111:1416–1418

Piper JM, Tonascia J, Matanoski GM (1985) Heavy phenacetin use and bladder cancer in women aged 20 to 49 years. N Engl J Med 313:292–295

Porpaczy P (1986) Phenacetinabusus – Verhältnisse in Österreich. In: Mihatsch MJ (ed) Das Analgetikasyndrom. Thieme, Stuttgart, pp 119–127

Pradalier A, Dry S, Baron JF (1984) Cephalée induite par l'abuse de tartrate d'ergotamine chez les migrainieux. Concours Méd 106:106–110

Rapaport A, Weeks R, Schaftell F (1985) Analgesic rebound headache: theoretical and practical implications. In: Olesen J, Tfelt-Hansen P, Jensen K (eds) Headache 85: Proceedings 2nd International Headache Congress, Copenhagen, pp 448–449

Rowsell AR, Neylan C, Wilkinson M (1973) Ergotamine induced headache in migrainous patients. Headache 13:65–67

Saper JR, Jones JM (1986) Ergotamine tartrate dependency: features and possible mechanisms. Clin Neuropharmacol 9:244–256

Schwarz A, Faber U, Glaeske G, Keller F, Oftermann G, Pommer W, Molzahn M (1985) Daten zu Analgetikakonsum und Analgetika-Nephropathie in der BRD. Öff Gesundheitswes 47:298–300

Spühler O, Zollinger HU (1950) Die chronisch interstitielle Nephritis. Helv Med Acta 17:564–567

Stewart JH (1978) Analgesic abuse and renal failure in Australia. Kidney Int 13:72–78

Tfelt-Hansen P (1985) Ergotamine headache. In: Pfaffenrath V, Lundberg PO, Sjaastad O (eds) Updating in headache. Springer, Berlin Heidelberg New York, pp 169–172

Tfelt-Hansen P, Krabbe AE (1981) Ergotamine abuse. Do patients benefit from withdrawal? Cephalalgia 1:29–32

Wainscott G, Volans G, Wilkinson M (1974) Ergotamine induced headaches. Br Med J ii:724

Wörz R (1983) Effects and risks of psychotropic and analgesic combinations. Am J Med 75:139–140

Wörz R, Baar H, Draf W, Garcia J, Gerbershagen HU, Gross D, Margin F, Ritter K, Scheifele J, Scholl W (1975) Kopfschmerz in Abhängigkeit von Analgetika-Mischpräparaten. Münch Med Wochenschr 177:457–462

Ergotism – The Clinical Picture

P. G. ANDERSSON

Introduction

The modern therapeutic use of ergotamine goes back to the 1930s, but the history of ergotamine goes back to the beginning of the European Middle Ages. Guggisberg (1954) and Wilkinson (1985) have described the use of ergotamine in detail. The poisonings in the Middle Ages and the placement of ergotamine in the cultural history of Europe have been described by Andersson (1982). Throughout the centuries epidemices of ignis infernalis have swept across Europe leaving thousands dead or crippled. Ergotism still exists, though the symptoms today are different in character and milder because ergotamine is now made synthetically in a pure form. Today the symptoms are caused mainly by wrong prescription of ergotamine to patients suffering from different types of headache. Ergotism is, however, very frequent. Andersson (1973) stated that 10% of headache patients in his clinic had ergotism symptoms. The picture has not changed to this day. Wilkinson (1985) reported that 4% of patients coming to the City of London Migraine Clinic in the years 1976–1981 had ergotism symptoms.

The clinical picture has been well described. Patients with chronic ergotism present many symptoms, all caused by the peripheral and central effects of ergotamine, but headache is the most frequent symptom. Thus the term "ergotamine headache" is very often synonymous with the fully developed clinical picture of ergotism as it will be in this paper. The aim of the present paper is to describe the clinical picture in patients who have a daily intake of ergotamine and to present some results of the treatment of such patients.

Material and Method

In the period from July 1985 to January 1986, 61 patients were diagnosed as having chronic daily headache and a daily consumption of ergotamine. All the patients used ergotamine as suppositories containing 2 mg ergotamine tartrate, 100 mg alisobumal, 100 mg caffeine, and 0.25 mg Bellafoline (Gynergen compound suppository). Of these 61 patients, 32 were followed up for more than 6 months after the first visit and the start of treatment to allow clarification of the course and control of the clinical picture after discontinuance of ergotamine. It is always difficult to determine what the original diagnosis was in patients who have abused medicines over several years. Out of the 32 patients followed up, 29

Hans Brogesvej 3 B, 8220 Brabrand, Denmark

Drug-Induced Headache
Ed. by H.-C. Diener and M. Wilkinson
© Springer-Verlag Berlin Heidelberg 1988

originally had headache attacks which could be characterized as common migraine while the remaining three patients probably had tension headache.

Table 1 shows the distribution according to sex and age. The duration of ergotamine abuse is shown in Table 2, and the daily ergotamine consumption in the last 2 months before the first visit is shown in Table 3. The main symptoms at the first visit are shown in Table 4.

The first phase in the treatment of these patients was to give them detailed information about ergotamine, caffeine, and barbiturates, and to tell them about the risk they expose themselves to if they continue the daily intake of ergotamine. Naturally all patients were informed about the transient deterioration of their headache which would occur when they stopped taking the drug. The information was combined with planning of the discontinuation. The patients were instructed how to use a warm knife to cut each suppository in half and to use only one half instead of a whole suppository. Most patients were able to do this, and, as a result, the intake of ergotamine tartrate was reduced by 50%. The second phase was treatment with tranquilizers while ergotamine was reduced further. Patients who were unable to accomplish this treatment on their own were offered hospitalization for 2–3 weeks for drug withdrawal therapy.

Table 1. Age and sex of 32 patients with ergotamine abuse

Age	Male	Female	Total
30–34	0	1	1
35–39	1	3	4
40–44	2	7	9
45–49	1	5	6
50–54	0	4	4
55–59	0	2	2
60–64	0	2	2
65–69	0	2	2
70 >=	0	2	2
Total	4	28	32

Table 2. Duration of ergotamine abuse in 32 patients

Duration (years)	Patients (n)
0– 2	2
3– 5	6
6– 8	5
9–11	10
12–14	3
15–17	1
18–20	3
>20	2

Table 3. The daily intake of ergotamine in 32 patients

Ergotamine (mg/day)	Patients (n)
1.0	9
1.5	4
2.0	5
2.5	3
3.0	2
3.5	2
4.0	6
4.5	0
5.0>	1

Table 4. The main symptoms in 32 patients with daily ergotamine consumption

Symptoms	Patients (n)
Cold feelings in hands and/or feet	10
Parestesia of hands and/or feet	10
Intermittent claudication	6
Spontaneous abortions (>2)	3
Nausea and/or vomiting	5
Tiredness	10
Depression	4
Daily headache	28
Withdrawal headache	24
No symptoms/without headache	5

Results of Discontinuance

After more than 6 months, 16 patients were free from ergotamine and barbiturates. None of these 16 patients had daily headaches and all their ergotism symptoms had disappeared. In nine of the 16 patients hospitalization was necessary. Of the remaining 16 patients seven were able to reduce ergotamine by 50% or more. The ergotism symptoms in these patients were less severe, particularly in patients with symptoms in the legs and feet. Headaches did not change enough to make any definite statement. In nine patients the daily ergotamine consumption and symptoms remained unchanged at follow-up. Among these nine patients four were free from ergotamine for about 2 months but then relapsed.

Discussion

Drug-induced headache is headache which develops during one or more types of medical treatment. It is important to add to such a definition that the headache must disappear when the medication is stopped. Most published papers state that drug-induced headache develops characteristically in adults, predominantly in women. Only a few papers mention that it is seen in children (Wilkinson 1985). Such a predominance in women cannot be explained only by the fact that headache is more common among women as the female/male ratio greater (28:4) than the one seen in a series of migraine patients (4 or 3:1). A vital role may be played by social, physiological, and psychological factors, but very little is known about such factors at present.

The results of treatment in such patients naturally varies with the type of treatment used. Relapses are commonly seen (Tfelt-Hansen and Krabbe 1981; Ala Hurula et al. 1982). It is interesting that in the paper by Tfelt-Hansen und Krabbe (1981) there were 11 patients who relapsed and that these patients were predominantly those who had been abusing ergotamine for 1 year or more. In the same paper there was an agreement between the patients' statements as to the amount of ergotamine used and the tracer (butalbital) in blood samples.

The type of ergotamine abuse varies from country to country. In Denmark practically all the abusers use suppositories and the abuse of tablets containing ergotamine is rare. This contradicts what is seen at the City of London Migraine Clinic. Such differences may be of importance as it seems to be more difficult to get patients using suppositories to stop them than it is those using tablets.

The developement of ergotamine and barbiturate abuse hardly differs from abuse of analgesics in headache patients. Initially the patient gets relief from headache and after months or years the patient starts to take ergotamine to avoid a headache which has not yet started. Gradually he or she takes ergotamine daily and the daily intake increases.

However other factors may be of importance, including social and psychological factors which at the moment, we know very little about. This is an item for research in the coming years.

References

Ala Hurula V, Myllylä V, Hokkanen E (1982) Ergotamine abuse: results of ergotamine discontinuation, with special reference to the plasma concentrations. Cephalalgia 2:189–195

Andersson PG (1973) Ergotamine headache. Headache 15:118–121

Andersson PG (1982) Medieval representations of cripples in the light of medical history. The Iconografic Post (Sweden), pp 6–13

Guggisberg H (1954) Vom Gift zum Heilstoff. Karger, Basel, pp 1–76

Tfelt-Hansen P, Krabbe AA (1981) Ergotamine abuse. Do patients benefit from withdrawal? Cephalalgia 1:29–32

Wilkinson M (1985) Ergotamine headache. In: Carrol JD, Pfaffenrath V, Sjaastad O (eds) Migraine and beta-blockade. Hässle, Mölndal

Clinical and Epidemiological Observations on Drug Abuse in Headache Patients

G. Micieli[1], G. C. Manzoni[2], F. Granella[2], E. Martignoni[1],
G. Malferrari[2], and G. Nappi[1]

Introduction

In recent years, the prophylactic treatment of primary headaches has been widely developed both in the theoretical and practical fields. New lines of drugs, non-pharmacological strategies and combined, sometimes highly effective approaches are responsible for this development. Nevertheless, despite the great number of controlled clinical trials on headache prophylaxis, similar approaches have not been provided in the management of the acute phase of headache. Thus, the chances of a successful outcome in this field are as limited as in the past. Treatment is restricted to the use of either ergotamine derivatives or various combination products, or nonsteroidal anti-inflammatory drugs which are widely used in many other painful conditions.

The prevailing opinions on the treatment of acute headache attacks have yielded a two-fold negative effect: first, only a few new pharmacological contributions have been directed toward the therapy of headache attacks; secondly, physicians usually give patients poor information regarding the most practical (and least dangerous) way to treat headache attacks. The result is that a great number of headache patients prescribe for themselves, on their own, various types of drugs and, as a consequence, analgesic overuse and abuse are frequently observed.

In fact, epidemiological data indicate that 75%–90% of the subjects taking analgesics do so without any medical prescription (Dunnel and Cartwright 1972).

In an epidemiological study conducted in Finland some years ago (Nikiforow 1980), 76% of the subjects suffering from headache took instant relief drugs; moreover, 27% of the headache patients took less then ten tablets per year, 32% more than ten tablets per year and less than ten per month, 17% more than ten per month.

Since the study was conducted on all the people who generally suffered from headache in the year prior to the survey (i.e., 70% of the Finnish population), it can be supposed that about 10% of these people take more than ten analgesic tablets per month for head pain. In the United Kingdom, Dunnel and Cartwright (1972) found that 41% of the adults interviewed had taken aspirin or other types of analgesics during the 2 weeks preceding the survey. In 50% of the cases they took analgesics to treat migraine or other forms of headache.

[1] Headache Centers, Department of Neurology, C. Mondino Foundation, University of Pavia, Via Palestro 3, 27100 Pavia, Italy
[2] Headache Center, Department of Neurology, University of Parma, Via del Quartiere 4, 43100 Parma, Italy

Drug-Induced Headache
Ed. by H.-C. Diener and M. Wilkinson
© Springer-Verlag Berlin Heidelberg 1988

Table 1. Nonprescription analgesics sold in Italy in 1985

	Units (*n*)
Aspirina (acidum acetylsalicylicum)	24 800 000
Optalidon (butalbitalum + propyphenazonum + coffeinum)	14 000 000
Saridon (propyphenazonum + paracetamolum + coffeinum)	9 000 000
Cibalgina (allobarbitalum + propyphenazonum)	7 700 000
Viamal (acidum acetylsalicylicum + coffeinum)	2 500 000
Mindol (racephedrinum + ethylmorphinum + coffeinum + propyphenazonum)	1 000 000

Furthermore, Saarela et al. (1975), in their investigation conducted in Finland, found that 19% of the people had taken analgesics without any medical prescription during the 2 days prior to the interview; in 57% of these cases they had taken analgesics because of headache. On the basis of recent investigations, more than 4% of the Swiss population abuses or is suspected of abusing drugs of various types; in 53% of the cases the drugs overused or abused are combination analgesics (Hornung and Gutsher 1984).

The corresponding data for the Italian population are not so recent; however, in 1985, 160 million units of non-narcotic analgesics were sold in Italy (i.e., over two per inhabitant) for an overall cost of about 110 million US dollars. Considering that more than 50% of the analgesics used (and abused) are taken for headache treatment, it may be reasonable to suppose that the cost for headache instant relief drugs is over 90 million US dollars. In particular, among the over-the-counter products, aspirin and combination products, such as Optalidon, Saridon, and Cibalgina, are the ones most frequently sold (Table 1). Indeed, the overall cost of analgesics is not high but this group of pain killers does not include the nonsteroidal anti-inflammatory compounds which are frequently also used in the acute treatment of headache because of their well-known analgesic properties. Thus, the overall cost for analgesics must also include this type of drug, of which about 50 million units per year are sold in Italy. It is evident, therefore, that, apart from the medical aspects, drug abuse is now so widespread as to represent a truly social and economical problem.

Since the most frequent reason for analgesic abuse appears to be headache, we carried out a retrospective epidemiological investigation over a 6-year period on the patients referred to the Headache Centers of the Parma and Pavia Universities in order to assess how many of them were drug abusers.

Subjects and Methods

In the absence of an international convention defining the concept of use and abuse of analgesics, we considered as drug abusers the patients who had taken instant-relief drugs every day for at least 1 year, regardless of the dosage. On the basis of this criterion, among 3000 consecutive patients referred to our Centers, 128 (4.3%) were found to be drug abusers; 32 of them were males and 96 females (Table 2); their ages ranged from 17 to 78 years (mean 45.4).

Table 2. Total population (1979–1985)

	Abusers		Nonabusers		Total	
	(n)	(%)	(n)	(%)	(n)	(%)
Males	32	3.9	782	96.1	814	100
Females	96	4.4	2090	95.6	2186	100
Total	128	4.3	2872	95.7	3000	100

The form of headache these patients were complaining of at the time of our first observation was identified using the diagnostic criteria of the Ad Hoc Committee on Classification of Headache (1962). However, this classification does not consider the temporal pattern of headache. Since all our patients had been suffering from daily chronic headache during at least the last year, we could classify them on the basis of a distinction between migraine, tension headache, and psychogenic forms of headache. In particular, we considered as suffering from migraine with interparoxysmal headache (MIH) the subjects with common migraine who over the years had developed headache between the migrainous attacks, which, in turn, had become more frequent, long-lasting and severe with reduced response to analgesics.

Moreover, patients with chronic tension headache (CTH) exhibited head pain which was either located on both sides of the back of the head and/or the forehead, or was of the "hood" type, generally nonthrobbing, rarely or never accompanied by signs of general or local impairment of the autonomic nervous system and associated with a "tensive" sensation (Sjaastad 1980; Nappi and Savoldi 1985). CTH may begin either with a daily chronic or episodic pattern, while MIH always appears as an episodic headache turning into a chronic form only later. The statistical analysis of the data was performed by the χ^2 method and Student's t test.

Results

Among the 128 subjects identified as abusers, 106 exhibited clinical features fitting the definition of MIH described above, while CTH was identified in 22 patients. As reported in Table 3, the sex distribution among CTH sufferers is quite different from that observed among MIH patients. CTH, in fact, appears equally among male and female abusers, while most of the MIH population is female, as in the episodic form of migraine.

The course of headache in our patients is reported in Table 4. Apart from a great variability, the most interesting finding is the very long period of time which is generally required for episodic migraine to turn into a chronic form of headache. By contrast, tension headache seems to acquire a chronic pattern earlier, so that the duration of the daily form of headache among CTH patients is significantly longer than in MIH sufferers.

Table 3. Distribution by sex and form of headache

	MIH		CTH		Total	
	(n)	(%)	(n)	(%)	(n)	(%)
Males	21	65.6	11	34.4	32	100
Females	85	88.5	11	11.5	96	100
Total	106	82.8	22	17.2	128	100

χ^2 test: $P < 0.01$.

Table 4. Course of headache

	MIH ($n=106$)	CTH ($n=22$)	Total ($n=128$)
Age at onset of episodic headache (years)	21.0	23.0	21.3
Age at transformation into daily chronic headache (years)	37.4	27.4	35.9
Duration of episodic headache (years)	16.4	11.0[b]	16.1
Duration of daily chronic headache (years)	5.9[a]	23.0[a]	8.5

[a] $P < 0.001$.
[b] 10 of the 22 patients suffer from secondary CTH.

Table 5. Possible factors favoring transformation of episodic headache into daily chronic headache (118 patients)

	(n)	(%)
Drug abuse	86	72.9
Arterial hypertension	12	10.2
Psychic trauma	11	9.3
Head injury	2	1.7
Inflammation of the skull and face	2	1.7
Surgically induced menopause	8/90	8.9
Childbirth	5/90	5.5
Early menopause	2/90	2.2
Non detectable factors	5	4.2

Moreover, considering all the factors that may be responsible for the transformation of an episodic into a chronic type of headache, we found out that the major cause is probably drug abuse itself, alone or associated with other less significant events (Table 5). Among the latter, drug abusers frequently reported arterial hypertension, psychic and head trauma. Among the female population either early or surgically induced menopause was considered a possible factor.

The mean duration of the daily intake of analgesics was 52.2 months, which is longer among CTH patients than in the MIH group, as is also suggested by the longer duration of the daily pattern. Moreover, in both the MIH and CTH pop-

Table 6. Duration of abuse

	MIH ($n=106$) (months)	CTH ($n=22$) (months)	Total ($n=128$) (months)
Males ($n=32$)	30.5	17.5	26.2
Females ($n=96$)	56.9	121.3	64.3
Total ($n=128$)	53.0	79.8	57.2

Table 7. Weekly amounts of instant relief drugs

Ergotamine-free analgesics (dose/week)	<10	10–20	>20	Mean
MIH	11[a]	15	32[a]	22.2
CTH	9[a]	5	2[a]	13.2
Total	20	20	34	
Ergotamine-containing analgesics (mg/week)	<10	10–24	>24	Mean
MIH	1	15	5	18.9

[a] χ^2 test: $P<0.01$.

ulations the duration of abuse was longer in females (Table 6). The weekly amount of instant relief drugs abused by our patients is reported in Table 7. Since ergotamine is a drug with peculiar pharmacological properties and with a limited range of use in headache in comparison to other instant relief drugs, it is reported separately, and its abuse is considered only for MIH patients.

The patients taking ergotamine-free drugs were divided into three groups:

1. Patients taking less than 10 doses (tablets and/or suppositories) per week
2. Patients taking between 10 and 20 doses per week
3. Patients taking more than 20 doses per week

Furthermore, ergotamine abusers were also divided into three groups on the basis of the weekly amount of active drug taken per week. Interestingly, most patients taking ergotamine-free drugs were heavy abusers (i.e., usually taking more than 20 doses per week), while in the ergotamine group patients more frequently appear to be "medium" abusers (between 10 and 20 doses per week). MIH patients took more ergotamine-free analgesics than those suffering from CTH and more frequently abused, at their first observation, only one type of analgesic (Table 8). Patients of both headache groups mostly abused the same type of analgesic over time without significant differences between MIH and CTH sufferers (Table 9).

When considering the chemical agents most commonly contained in the instant relief drugs abused by our patients, it can be seen that caffeine is taken by almost all patients, ergotamine by about a quarter of them and morphine-like substances by less than 10% (Table 10). As to the type of drug abused, it emerges

Table 8. Drugs abused at patient's first observation

	MIH ($n=106$)		CTH ($n=22$)		Total ($n=128$)	
	(n)	(%)	(n)	(%)	(n)	(%)
Only one type	88	83.0	11	50.0	99	77.3
Two or more types	18	17.0	11	50.0	29	22.7

χ^2 test: $P<0.01$.

Table 9. Drugs abused over time

	MIH ($n=106$)		CTH ($n=22$)		Total ($n=128$)	
	(n)	(%)	(n)	(%)	(n)	(%)
Always the same type	86	81.1	18	81.8	104	81.2
Previous abuse of different types	20	18.9	4	18.2	24	18.8

Table 10. Chemical agents

	Patients	
	(n)	(%)
Caffeine	111	86.7
Pyrazolone derivatives	91	71.1
Barbiturates	60	46.9
Ergotamine	31	24.2
Para-aminophenol derivatives	28	21.9
Indomethacin	16	12.5
Phenothiazines	16	12.5
Opiates	12	9.4
Salicylates	10	7.8
Others	33	25.7

that when MIH and CTH patients are compared, the MIH group frequently abuses Optalidon, a combination analgesic containing butalbital and caffeine, while ergotamine abuse is limited to 28.3% of MIH cases and to one single patient suffering from CTH (Table 11).

Combination products are also preferred by the CTH group which uses Optalidon and Saridon (containing propyphenazon, paracetamol and caffeine) widely. Other over-the-counter products appear to be less frequently abused among CTH patients; however, the abuse of these products is significantly higher when compared with that of MIH subjects. On the other hand, CTH and MIH patients also show obvious differences in drug intake when other types of products are considered (Table 12). CTH patients are, in fact, found to abuse anxyo-

Table 11. Type of drugs

	MIH ($n=106$)		CTH ($n=22$)		Total ($n=128$)		χ^2 test P value
	(n)	(%)	(n)	(%)	(n)	(%)	
Optalidon	37	34.9	8	36.4	45	35.2	NS
Ergotamine[a]	30	28.3	1	4.5	31	24.2	<0.05
Saridon	18	17.0	10	45.4	28	21.9	<0.01
Difmetre	11	10.4	5	22.7	16	12.5	NS
Opiates	7	6.6	5	22.7	12	9.4	<0.05
Aspirina[a]	5	4.7	5	22.7	10	7.8	<0.02
Novalgina[a]	5	4.7	5	22.7	10	7.8	<0.02
Others	4	3.8	2	9.1	6	4.7	NS

[a] Monosubstances.

Table 12. Abuse of drugs other than analgesics

	MIH ($n=106$)		CTH ($n=22$)		Total ($n=128$)	
	(n)	(%)	(n)	(%)	(n)	(%)
Anxyolitics and/or sleep inducers	13[a]	12.3	15[a]	68.2	28	21.9
Laxatives	11	10.4	3	13.6	14	10.9
None	82[a]	77.3	4[a]	18.2	86	67.2

[a] χ^2 test: $P<0.001$.

litics and/or sleep inducers (which are probably prescribed to them for problems other than headache) more frequently than the subjects suffering from MIH.

Discussion

Despite the common opinion that analgesic abuse and related drug-induced headache are more frequently sustained by ergotamine consumption, and in contrast with a recent epidemiological study carried out in the Federal Republic of Germany by Dichgans et al. (1984; see also Peters and Horton 1951; Hokkanen et al. 1978; Lucas and Falkowsky 1973; Rowsell et al. 1973), our data indicate that headache sufferers can become abusers of any instant relief drug, as is proven by the fact that the over-the-counter drugs sold most in Italy are at the top of the list of the most widely abused patented medications. In contrast to other recent investigations, our study also indicates a lower incidence of ergotamine abusers in comparison to data previously reported by other authors (Isler 1982; Kudrow 1982; Mathew et al. 1987).

This fact may be ascribed to the widespread practice of deciding for oneself the treatment with the most popular combination products sold in Italy, and it is noteworthy that drugs containing ergotamine, and in many cases barbiturates, are available in Italy only on prescription.

Moreover, the possible failure of the general practitioners to indentify correctly the exact form of primary headache complained of by their patients could also explain the limited number of ergotamine abusers we found among our patients. The more frequent finding of "medium" abusers might be explained by a self-limiting side effect mechanism which ergotamine will easily sustain.

Furthermore, when headache acquires a chronic pattern which is often favored by the very abuse of analgesics, the diagnostic problems become more important. In our experience all the patients found to be drug abusers suffered from a chronic form of headache, with great differences among MIH and CTH patients in type and daily dosage of the drug abused, onset of abuse in respect to headache onset, and, finally, looking for other types of pharmacological substances.

Moreover, in contrast with other surveys (Langemark and Olesen 1984) the incidence of abusers of morphine-like substances is very low among our patients, with a slight prevalence in the CTH group. On the other hand, almost half of the drugs abused by our patients contain barbiturates which have been known for a long time to induce addiction and chronic headache. An even greater number of our patients consumed caffeine, which the Ad Hoc Committee had already considered as capable of inducing headache.

These observations, however, do not seem to clarify the controversial question of whether analgesics may transform episodic headache into a chronic form. We found that analgesic abuse is often reported as concomitant with this modification in the temporal pattern of headache, while neuroendocrine and neurophysiological investigations seem to support the view that, at least for migraine, the acquisition of a chronic pattern associated with ever more serious abuse of analgesics may depend on the progressive deterioration of the pain control system (Genazzani et al. 1984; Nappi et al. 1985). Additional studies, psychobiological, neurophysiological, and neuropharmacological in particular, are necessary to define exactly the nature of the more and more widespread failure of adaptive processes in response to environmental stimuli characterizing these patients and to identify a correct therapeutic strategy for the management of these chronic forms of headache.

Moreover, in Italy adequate changes in the health system, based on educational programs for patients and general practitioners, as well as on more severe restrictions on the sale of the over-the-counter medications, seem to be desirable to limit analgesic abuse among headache sufferers.

Summary

Among 3000 consecutive patients referred to our Headache Centers, 4.3% were found to be drug abusers, having taken instant relief drugs every day for at least 1 year. The presenting type of headache was migraine with interparoxysmal headache (MIH) in 82.8% and chronic tension headache (CTH) in 17.2% of the cases. Almost all patients were abusers of several analgesics and the average duration of daily intake was 52.2 months. Most of the patients taking ergotamine-free drugs were heavy abusers; by contrast, among the patients taking ergotamine the majority were "medium" abusers. Our data indicate that headache sufferers can become abusers of any instant relief drug and that no significant differences exist between ergotamine and other drugs as potential factors "favoring abuse." Finally, in our patients drug abuse was also found to be the biggest single factor favoring the transformation of episodic into daily chronic headache.

References

Ad Hoc Committee on Classification of Headache of the NIH (1962). JAMA 179:717–718

Dichgans J, Diener HC, Gerber WD, Verspohl EJ, Kukiolka H, Kluck M (1984) Analgetika-induzierter Dauerkopfschmerz. Dtsch Med Wochenschr 109:369–373

Dunnel K, Cartwright A (1972) Medicine takers, prescribers and hoarders. Routledge and Kegan, London

Genazzani AR, Nappi G, Facchinetti F, Micieli G, Petraglia F, Bono G, Monittola C, Savoldi F (1984) Progressive impairment of CSF B-EP levels in migraine sufferers. Pain 18:127–133

Hokkanen E, Waltimo O, Kallaranta T (1978) Toxic effects of ergotamine used for migraine. Headache 18:95–98

Hornung G, Gutscher H (1984) Medikamentenabusus: Ergebnisse einer Repräsentativerhebung in der deutschsprachigen Schweiz. Drogalkohol (Lausanne) 8:3–24

Isler H (1982) Migraine treatment as a cause of chronic migraine. In: Rose FC (ed) Advances in migraine research and therapy. Raven, New York, pp 159–164

Kudrow L (1982) Paradoxical effects of frequent analgesic use. In: Critchley M, Friedman AP, Gorini S, Sicuteri F (eds) Advances in neurology, vol 33. Raven, New York, pp 335–341

Langemark M, Olesen J (1984) Drug abuse in migraine patients. Pain 19:81–86

Lucas RN, Falkowsky W (1973) Ergotamine and methysergide abuse in patients with migraine. Br J Psychiatry 122:199–203

Mathew NT, Reuveni U, Perez F (1987) Transformed or evolutive migraine. Headache 27:102–106

Nappi G, Savoldi F (1985) Headache. Diagnostic system and taxonomic criteria. Libbey, London

Nappi G, Facchinetti F, Martignoni E, Petraglia F, Manzoni GC, Sances G, Sandrini G, Genazzani AR (1985) Endorphin patterns within the headache spectrum disorders. Cephalalgia 5 [Suppl 2]:201–210

Nikiforow R (1980) Headache medication habits in northern Finland. Headache 20:274–278

Peters GA, Horton BT (1951) Headache: with special reference to the excessive use of ergotamine preparations and withdrawal effects. Mayo Clin Proc 26:153–161

Rowsell AR, Neylan C, Wilkinson M (1973) Ergotamine-induced headaches in migrainous patients. Headache 13:65–67

Saarela S, Yrjölä M, Isokoski M (1975) Consumption of self-selected drugs. Suomen Jääk 30:29–33

Sjaastad O (1980) So-called "tension headache": a term in need of revision? Curr Med Res Opin 6:41–54

Drug-Induced Headache –
Does a Critical Dosage Exist?

E. Scholz, H.-C. Diener, and S. Geiselhart

Introduction

Although the clinical problem of chronic daily headache induced by chronic intake of ergotamine tartrate and/or analgesics is known to clinicians (Lippman 1955; Horton et al. 1963; Rowsell et al. 1973; Wainscott et al. 1974; Andersson 1975; Ala-Hurula et al. 1982; Kudrow 1982; Saper 1983; Dichgans et al. 1984), no information is as yet available about the dosages of different drugs necessary to provoke this response. The patients' histories show a gradual increase in frequency and dose of drug intake, eventually ending in daily administration of high dosages. It is unknown whether the daily intake itself or the drug dosage plays the crucial role.

With ergotamine tartrate, it took a long time to learn about the conditions leading to headache since early studies were not even able to detect ergotamine in blood samples, although clinical effects were observable (see Tfelt-Hansen 1982 and this volume). Surprisingly, different analgesics and secale alkaloids, including ergotamine tartrate and dihydroergotamine derivatives, with quite different pharmacological properties induce headaches which are clinically similar or even identical (Isler 1982; Kudrow 1982; Saper 1983; Dichgans et al. 1984). Whereas ergotamine tartrate is known to exert long-lasting effects on blood vessels, probably resulting in a prolonged vasoconstriction (Tfelt-Hansen 1986) and thus inducing "vascular" headache, the pathophysiology of drug-induced headache is still completely unknown. It is tempting to speculate on the role of prostaglandin, vasopressin, and kinins, substances known to alter the sensitivity of vascular smooth muscles (Saxena 1982). Another possible mechanism is muscle tension. We have as yet no explanation why a great number of patients complain about intensive pain in the neck musculature during and shortly after withdrawal.

We have tried to investigate possible causes and risks of analgesic drug consumption by analyzing what dosages of particular drugs or drug combinations were able to induce chronic headache and then comparing these dosages with the usual intake in migraine patients without chronic headache.

Department of Neurology, University of Tübingen, Liebermeisterstr. 18–20, 7400 Tübingen, Federal Republic of Germany

Drug-Induced Headache
Ed. by H.-C. Diener and M. Wilkinson
© Springer-Verlag Berlin Heidelberg 1988

Patients and Methods

Migraine Patients

Data on the drug intake in 61 migraine patients were collected prospectively. We used the diary data of patients who were to join a study for prophylactic migraine treatment. In an 8-week baseline period before the start of prophylactic treatment, patients were instructed to take their abortive medication as usual and to register drugs, migraine duration, migraine days, and concomitant headaches, but to avoid prophylactic drugs like beta-blockers and calcium channel blockers. None of them had daily or near daily headache.

The dose of each different substance taken was calculated from these data and the intake per month estimated. The overall dosage during the 4-week period was calculated as intake per month. The intake per month was divided by the headache days, which were similar to the days with drug intake, in order to estimate the mean daily intake per headache day for each single substance.

This group was subdivided into subgroups (group 1) with 1–9 headache days per month (mean 5.2 days, SD 2.3 days) and an "at risk" group (group 2) with 10 and more headache days (mean 12.2 days, SD 2.1 days). Our hypothesis was that group 2 patients would show the development or a tendency to a higher drug intake compared to group 1 and thus be at an intermediate stage on the way to chronic daily headache. As shown in Table 1, patients with migraine (groups 1 and 2) showed approximately the same male:female ratio and the same mean age as patients with chronic daily headache (3:1).

Chronic Daily Headache Patients

A total of 39 patients with daily drug-induced headache were treated on an inpatient basis by strict withdrawal of all analgesic drugs. Their drug intake was evaluated retrospectively. Our operational definition of this group (group 3) was that patients should report headache every day over a time period of at least 1 year. On their 1st day in the clinic, they underwent a standardized interview about their previous drug intake behavior. They were questioned about the drugs, the mean and maximum daily intake, their overall intake during the last 14 days, the duration of their chronic headache and drug abuse, and the different drugs they had been taking in their medical history. Furthermore, they were questioned about the specific headache symptoms and whether or not changes in symptomatology had taken place in order to clarify when chronic daily headache had started. From their overall mean daily intake, we calculated the monthly and daily intake of chemically defined substances. Since most patients took tablets as well as suppositories in varying amounts, we calculated the overall dosage without specifying the route of administration. We are well aware of the fact that the route of administration is important as the uptake is greater rectally than orally. Demographic data of the patients are given in Table 1.

The final diagnosis of the primary headache in patients with chronic daily headache was made using the biographic data and the outcome of drug with-

Table 1. Demographic data of 39 patients with chronic headache and 68 patients with migraine

Chronic headache	Migraine
Patients	
n 39	68
Female 31	51
Male 8	17
Age (years)	
Mean 42.6	42.8
SD 13.5	9.7
History of chronic headache (years)	
Mean 6.6	
SD 6.9	
Range 0.5–25	

drawal. Thus, 29 of the patients initially suffered from common migraine, five from tension headache, one each from post-traumatic headache, hypotonia, and depression. In two patients no distinct diagnosis of primary headache was possible.

Statistical Analysis

We calculated the mean and median dosages of intake per headache day and per month for each single drug. For group comparisons we used a median as the basis since the values within the groups were not normally distributed. For group comparisons we therefore used nonparametric tests (Mann-Whitney Wilcoxon).

Results

Overall Consumption Characteristics (Table 2)

All 39 patients with drug-induced headache used fixed combinations of drugs, none of them took remedies containing only one substance. A total of 27 patients took combinations including ergot derivatives, the remaining 12 used different combinations of analgesics (mainly salicylic acid = aspirin and/or acetaminophen = paracetamol combined with caffeine) without any ergot derivatives. Due to the fact that a number of migraine drugs and even analgesics on the market in the Federal Republic of Germany at the time of the study still contained barbiturates, 14 patients used combinations including different barbiturate derivatives (butalbital, pentobarbital, phenobarbital), these are taken together and referred to here as "barbiturates." An additional abuse of benzodiazepines (diazepam, bromazepam, oxacepam, camazepam) was observed in five patients.

Table 2. Drug consumption characteristics in 39 patients with chronic headache

	(n)
Drug combinations	39
Pure analgesics	0
Including	
Ergotamine tartrate	15
Dihydroergotamine	14
Both	2
Barbiturates	14
Benzodiazepines	5
Different combinations of analgesics without ergots	12

Intake of Different Substances

When groups 1 (less than 10 migraine days) and 3 (chronic daily headache) were compared, the overall drug intake per month and the cumulative dosages of all substances were significantly higher in group 3 (see Table 3). This result is self-explanatory. Surprisingly, the median and mean intake per month in group 2 (10 and more headache days per month) did not differ from the intake in group 1. We had expected an increase of dosages toward the values of the chronic group. However, group 2 is small for all substances so that these results have to be considered with caution.

The median intake of salicylic acid and acetaminophen of 49 and 33 g per month with a maximum intake of 86 and 130 g per month, respectively, showed the exorbitant amount of analgesics taken in chronic headache. When the chronic headache group was subdivided into subgroups taking combination of analgesics with and without ergotderivatives, no significant difference was found in the dosages of analgesics per month or per day.

Ergotamine Tartrate (Figs. 1 and 2)

The maximum intake of ergotamine tartrate per month in groups 1 and 2 was 24 mg. This fits quite well with earlier recommendations to limit the dose per month to 24 mg (Wilkinson 1983). Only one patient in group 3 took less than 24 mg per month (7 mg). To be even safer, the dose per month could be limited to 10 mg corresponding to the median intake in the migraine group. The maximal daily intake (4 mg) in group 1 again fitted well with the recommendation of limiting the daily dose to 4 mg. The median daily intake of abusers, however, accounted for only 3.4 mg, which is below the limit, and ten of the 15 patients with chronic daily headache took less than 4 mg per day.

Table 3. Drug intake per month

Substance	Migraine group 1			Migraine group 2			Chronic daily headache			Migraine group 1 vs. chronic group 3 Mann-Whitney Wilcoxon test (P)
	(n)	Median dose (mg)	Dose range (mg)	(n)	Median dose (mg)	Dose range (mg)	(n)	Median dose (mg)	Dose range (mg)	
Ergotamine tartrate	20	5.85	0.7–24	5	8.0	4–25	15	84.0	7–294	<0.01
Dihydro-ergotamine	14	6.0	0.5–20	2	11.7	3.5–20	14	63.0	14–277	<0.01
Phenazone	25	1025.0	200–4800	3	1500	875–6500	15	14000.0	3500–42000	<0.001
Salicylic acid	19	2050.0	225–7400	2	4000	3500–4500	14	49000.0	500–86000	<0.001
Acetaminophen	21	1600.0	400–4400	5	3700.0	1500–13000	21	33600.0	11200–130200	<0.001
Caffeine	45	450.0	50–1460	9	800	125–2600	38	8400	1120–29400	<0.001
Codeine	14	125.0	10–630	3	200.0	115–430	14	980.0	280–5600	<0.001
Barbiturates	32	250.0	30–1200	6	500.0	200–1250	14	4200.0	1000–14000	<0.001

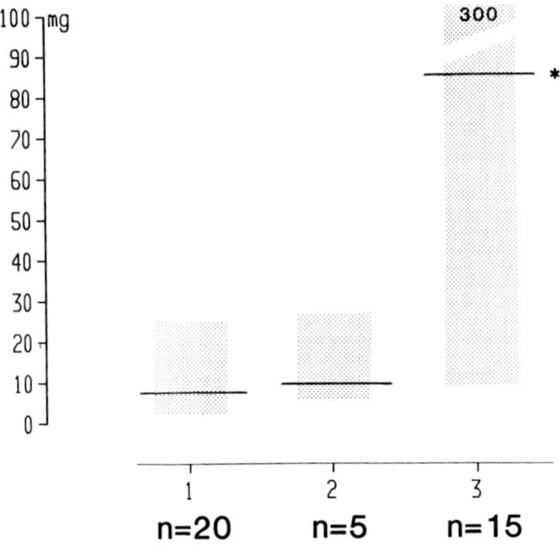

Fig. 1. The ergotamine intake per month is shown for the different groups of headache patients (for detailed description see Patients and Methods). *1*, group 1: patients with less than 10 headache days per month; *2*, group 2: patients with more than 10 headache days per month; *3*, group 3 with chronic daily headache. The *bar* indicates the median value for the groups, the *shaded area* indicates the overall range. The numbers of patients in the groups are indicated below the group specification. The difference between group 1 and 3 is significant (Mann-Whitney Wilcoxon test for nonparametric group comparisons; * $P<0.05$; ** $P<0.01$; *** $P<0.001$)

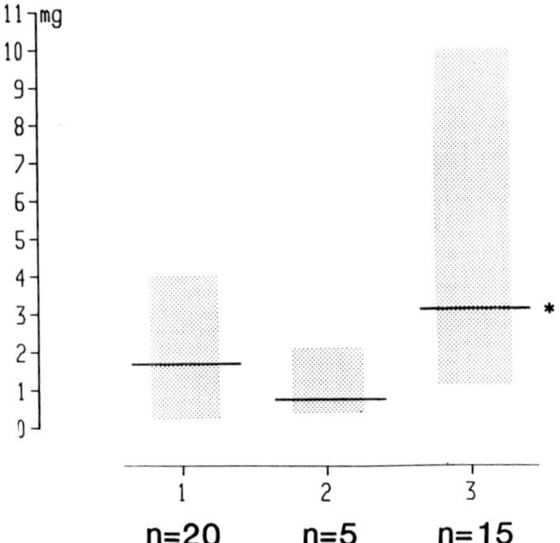

Fig. 2. The ergotamine intake per day is shown. See Fig. 1 for explanation of symbols

Dihydroergotamine (Figs. 3 and 4)

The chronic intoxication by ergotamine is well documented. However, little if anything, is known about the role of dihydrated ergot derivatives when chronically administred. In our sample dihydroergotamine (DHE) was involved in chronic headache as often as ergotamine (14 versus 15 patients). The mean dose per month in group 3 was comparable to that of ergotamine (99.8 mg versus 102.5 mg), the median even lower (63.0 versus 84.0), so that comparable effects of chronically applied DHE may be suspected. Calculating the daily dosage, there was again a similar mean value (DHE 3.56 mg versus ergotamine 3.42 mg) and an even lower median value (DHE 2.25 mg versus ergotamine 3.0 mg).

Another line of evidence that DHE is able to induce or add to the induction of chronic headache can be deduced from our experience with DHE in migraine prophylaxis. Thirteen patients were treated with 10 mg DHE per day over

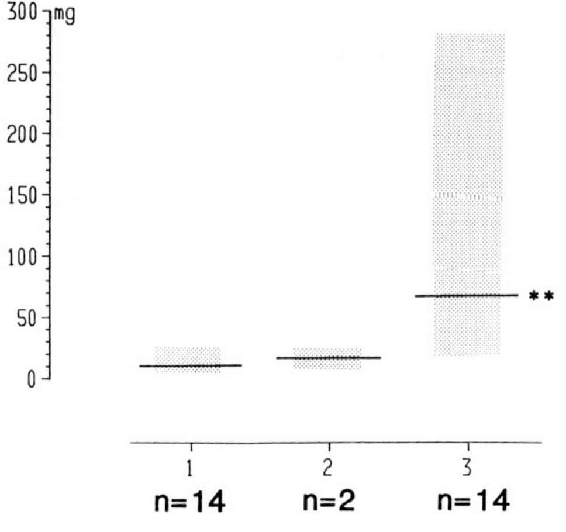

Fig. 3. Dihydroergotamine intake per month. See Fig. 1 for explanation of symbols

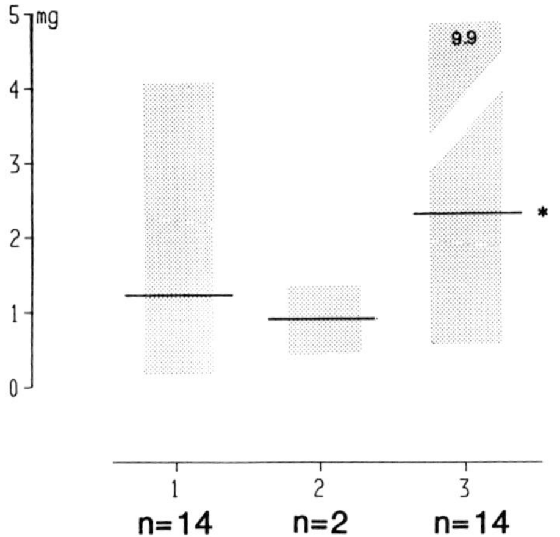

Fig. 4. Dihydroergotamine intake per day. See Fig. 1 for explanation of symbols

4 months and 5 mg per day for a further 3 months. Of these patients, 30% responded to therapy and showed a decrease in migraine frequency. The duration of concomitant headache (but not of migraine attacks), however, increased during long-term treatment. During month 5 of treatment, headache duration increased by 80% in month 6 by 115% above baseline levels (see Fig. 5).

Phenazone, Acetaminophen, and Salicylic Acid

The two pyrazolone derivatives, phenazone and propyphenazone, were summarized under the heading "phenazone." They are analgesics and antipyretics with an efficacy comparable to salicylates. They are only (but in the Federal Republic of Germany widely) used in analgesic mixtures together with sedatives, antihistaminics, and opioides like codeine. The intake per month showed a median of 14 g

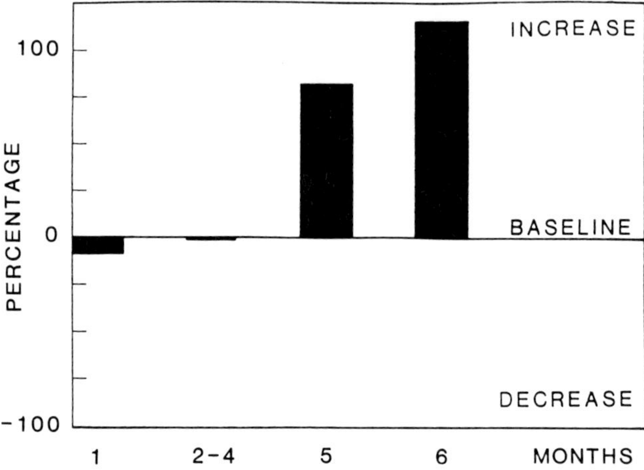

Fig. 5. The headache duration in prophylactic treatment with DHE in a group of migraine patients is plotted as the percentage of the headache duration during an 8-week baseline period. The study is explained in more detail in Results. An initial minor decrease in headache duration during month 1 of treatment changes into a considerable increase in headache duration in months 5 and 6. This effect is interpreted as indicating the development of headache under chronic intake of DHE

and a maximum of 42 g. The median intake per day and per month was lower by a factor of 2–3 than comparable data on acetaminophen and salicylic acid. The daily intake as well as the intake per month were significantly increased in group 3.

Data concerning daily dosages of acetaminophen and salicylic acid are strikingly similar (see Figs. 6 and 7). In group 3, the median dosages were 1200 and 1500 mg, respectively. This fits well with their similar analgesic potency and can be used as a hint that the headache-inducing effects might depend on similar pharmacological mechanisms. The high median and maximum dosages per month in

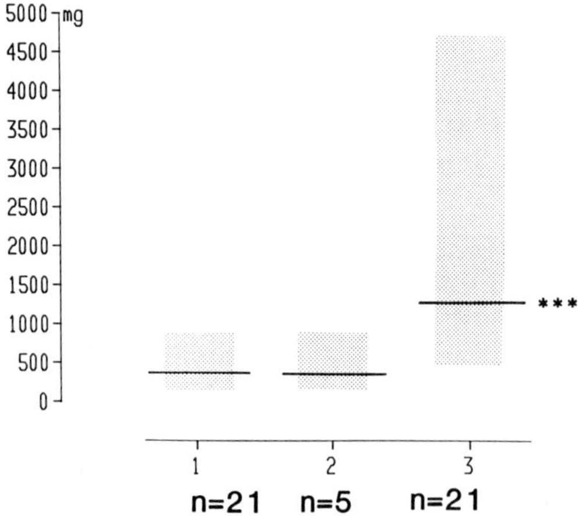

Fig. 6. Acetaminophen intake per month. See Fig. 1 for explanation of symbols

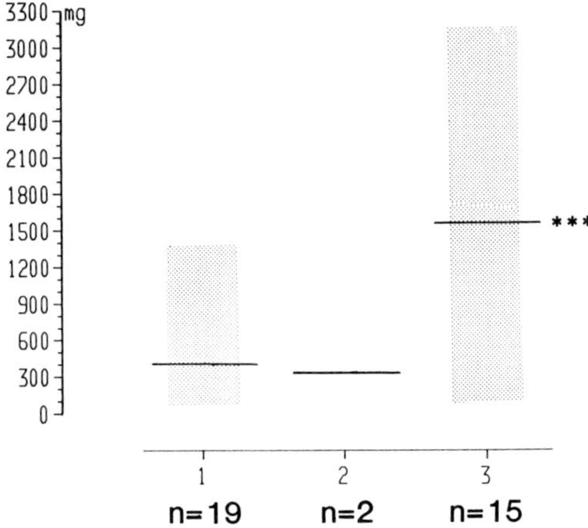

Fig. 7. Salicylic acid intake per day. See Fig. 1 for explanation of symbols

group 3 for both substances point to their role in the induction of systemic side effects like nephropathy with papillary necrosis and chronic interstitial nephritis.

Caffeine

Since caffeine is included in most of the antimigraine drugs and analgesics in the Federal Republic of Germany, it was inevitably taken by most of our migraine patients (53 of 68) and by all but one of the chronic headache patients. Again, the dosages of daily intake and intake per month were significantly increased in chronic headache patients.

Codeine

In contrast to all other drugs in the study, the codeine consumption on a daily basis was not significantly increased in the abuse group. This is especially interesting in the discussion on the role of codeine as a drug which potentially leads to addiction.

Barbiturates

Barbiturates are still widely used in migraine drugs in the Federal Republic of Germany as shown by 38 group 1 and 2 patients, and 14 group 3 patients. Yet the percentage of patients in the "nonaddiction group" is higher than in the chronic headache "addiction group" (55% versus 36%). The mean and median daily intake is, however, considerably higher in group 3 and again significantly higher than in the migraine group (see Fig. 8).

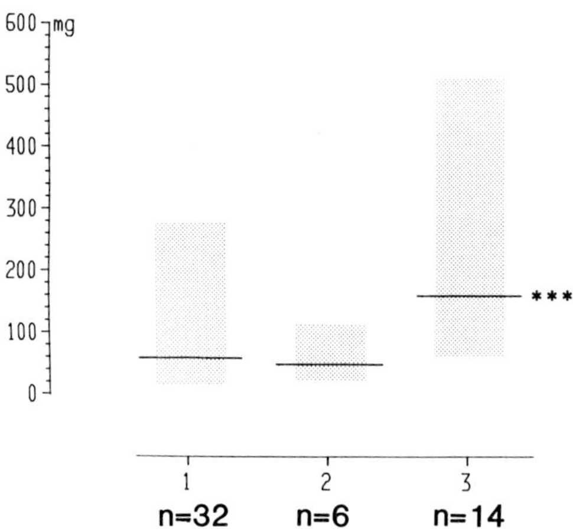

Fig. 8. Barbiturate intake per day. See Fig. 1 for explanation of symbols

Discussion

It is evident from our study that all patients with chronic headache consumed migraine and headache drugs more frequently and in higher dosages than migraine patients without chronic headache. One might argue that this behavior is a logical consequence of frequent headache. The fact, however, that this kind of headache improves dramatically after drug intake is stopped (see Diener et al., this volume) supports our explanation that this kind of headache is caused by drug abuse.

The interpretation of our data is crucial in one important aspect: most of the patients were taking more than one substance at a time since migraine remedies and so-called pain killers on the market contain a variety of substances (combination drugs). The usefulness of most if not all of these combined drugs has been under debate for many years. For simplification, we calculated the data for each single substance as if these were single drugs.

We are aware of a second important objection: that it is not the daily dosage but rather the continuous daily drug intake which causes chronic headache. The pharmacological experience with ergotamine demonstrates that in addition to daily intake a critical amount of biologically active substance has to be consumed. In the meantime, the pharmacokinetic effects of ergotamine have been well investigated (see Tfelt-Hansen, this volume and 1986). The effects of 0.5 mg ergotamine tartrate intravenously and 2–4 mg of a single rectal dose on parameters of vascular compliance (toe-arm systolic gradient) are comparable. Repetitive doses of 2–4 mg ergotamine are thus capable of inducing chronic vasoconstriction. This fits well with the mean daily dose of 3.4 mg ergotamine tartrate which our chronic headache group had been taking. We therefore believe that our way of calculating "dosages at risk" might in an analogous way throw some light on the effects of other substances.

DHE has been reported to increase preferentially the tone of veins (Aellig 1982, 1984). In acute experiments, 1 mg DHE i.v. (and 0.5 mg ergotamine i.v.) did not change cerebral blood flow, and acute vasoconstrictory effects on cerebral vessels could not be observed (Tfelt-Hansen 1986). This has been interpreted as a missing effect of acutely administred DHE on cerebral arteries. However, alkaloids like dihydroergotoxine and DHE are bound to tissue and are then slowly eliminated with a long terminal half-life of 22 h (Woodcock et al. 1982; Linblad et al. 1983). Although DHE is a less potent vasoconstrictor than ergotamine, it does exert an intrinsic vasoconstrictor action (Müller-Schweinitzer and Fanchamps 1982). On the other hand, DHE inhibits, as a competitive inhibitor, the alpha-adrenergic effects on cranial and peripheral arteries, and, as a noncompetitive antagonist, the 5-hydroxytryptamine effects, thus making these vessels less responsive to systemic influences. The functional role of different DHE metabolites is not yet understood (Aellig 1984; Maurer and Frick 1984). These active metabolites might play an additional role in the chronic effects of DHE.

Earlier clinical observers reported that not only ergotamine but also DHE were abused to the same extent by patients with chronic headache (Isler 1982; Dichgans et al. 1984). Our data from this study and from the prospective treatment with DHE (see Results) suggest that a chronic intake of 3–4 mg DHE is able to induce increased and, finally, chronic headache despite a decrease in the number of migraine attacks. This means that the chronic effects of DHE and ergotamine both occur with doses of 3–4 mg per day. We therefore suggest that the long-term effects of DHE on the vascular sensitivity should be investigated in order to confirm these findings.

While data and knowledge on ergotamine-induced headache has grown considerably, little, if anything, is known about headache induced by analgesics. Not only do ergotamine- and DHE-containing combination drugs induce headache, but also analgesics such as acetaminophen and salicylic acid have been accused of inducing chronic headache (Isler 1982; Langemark and Olesen 1984; Mathew 1982 and this volume; Henry et al. 1985). The reported incidence of abuse of analgesics alone seems to be lower than that of analgesics in combination with ergotamine. Twelve out of 39 patients, who were taking analgesics only (acetaminophen or salicylic acid in combination with each other and/or caffeine) was considerably more than the nine out of 90 patients reported by Langemark and Olesen (1984). Only one really large group taking analgesics (90 patients) has been reported (Rapoport et al. 1985). Rapoport et al. described the development of "rebound headache":

While small amounts of analgesics offer some relief in scalp muscle contraction headache initially, individuals with frequent pain seem to habituate to the therapeutic actions of such agents. This begins a cycle of increased intake to achieve similar relief. At some point, increased consumption not only fails to provide pain reduction but it begins to perpetuate and intensify headache.

Their patients were consuming an average of 34.5 analgesic tablets per week, they did not, however, report on the average dosage of the involved substances. These five tablets per day with the usual amount (in the United States) of 325 mg acetaminophen and 200–350 mg salicylic acid per tablet amount to an average of 1000–1600 mg of these analgesics, an amount similar to that reported by us. One important point is that on the market in the Federal Republic of Germany, minor analgesics are often freely available in combination drugs containing both acetaminophen and salicylic acid, usually combined with caffeine. Patients taking analgesics only therefore often took the median salicylic acid plus 1200 mg acetaminophen. With dosages of 300–600 mg, the salicylate half-life in adults is about 3 h. Under normal circumstances, there is no risk of cumulation. A small increase in dose, however, results in a disproportionate rise in plasma salicylate concentrations since with large doses the conjugation with glycine and the formation of salicyluric acid is saturated, and the half-life increases to 20–40 h (Gibson et al. 1975). High dosages might therefore lead to cumulation. Since a toxic over-dosage of salicylic acid may lead to cerebral edema, effects on cerebral blood flow vessels can be postulated, probably even in lower dosages.

Other antipyretics, such as indomethacine are known to cause headache in 20%–60% of patients (Suihovec 1980), showing these potential side effects in other drugs with action on the prostaglandin synthesis. Since phenazone is contained only in combination drugs including ergotamine, DHE, and acetaminophen, the lower mean dose of this minor analgesic does not reflect its real risk. From its analgesic efficacy one would have expected dosages in the range of those taken by salicylic acid and acetaminophen. According to our results, acetaminophen and salicylic acid are not only equipotent and equianalgesic on a weight basis (Beaver 1981), but also equipotent in the ability to produce chronic headache. Our data suggest that in chronic intake, dosages of more than 1000 mg per day are able to induce chronic headache syndromes.

There is much discussion about the effects of caffeine in combination with analgesics. While Woodbury and Fingl (1975) state that in controlled trials analgesic mixtures containing caffeine have not been found to be superior to salicylic acid for the relief of headache, Laska et al. (1984) concluded that caffeine increased the effects of analgesics by 40%. Our chronic headache patients reported a mean intake of about 300 mg caffeine per day, equivalent to three to four cups of coffee. The intake of this amount of caffeine leads to an increase in systolic and diastolic blood pressure with a decreased heart rate due to a progressive increase in systemic vascular resistance (Pincomb et al. 1985). This again indicates the direct vascular effects of chronic caffeine consumption, although the effects on cerebral circulation of chronic caffeine intake and sudden withdrawal are unknown (Mathew and Wilson 1985). The effects of caffeine on headache vary depending on the dose. Excessive dosages of caffeine are known to produce headache; the same is true of withdrawal (Mathew and Wilson 1985). Single doses can lead to an improvement of headache (Bruce et al. 1986). The withdrawal headache which occurs after cessation of caffeine intake and the psychotropic effects of caffeine might contribute to the abuse of combination drugs (Mathew et al. 1982; Dichgans et al. 1984). The overall intake of 300 mg in our chronic headache group, however, seems to be only a moderate dosage since 20%–30% of a normal population report a consumption of more than 500–600 mg caffeine per day (Mathew and Wilson 1985).

The role of barbiturates, and especially of those with short action in drug addiction, is well known and will not be discussed here in detail. Our data show a clear increase in dosage of barbiturates in patients with chronic daily headache, most of them taking up to 500 mg per day. We had expected the same effects for the opioid derivative codeine. However, it was the only drug which was not taken in significantly increased dosage in chronic daily headache. The mean daily dose of 50 mg in our patient group is within the therapeutic range of 10–60 mg (Babayan et al. 1980; Meadows 1984). We have no really satisfactory explanation for this difference, which might be due to the relatively low addiction potential of codeine (Meadows 1984). In contrast to barbiturates, codeine has intrinsic analgesic effects and is known to enhance the effects of minor analgesics (Meadows 1984).

One common observation in all but one of the abused drugs was the significant increase in daily intake, one of the known characteristics of addiction in general. This might in part be explained by the fact that many of the drugs were used in fixed combinations. However this effect cannot be related to any single drug, neither to ergot derivatives nor to minor analgesics or sedatives. All of these drugs or drug combinations seem to be able to produce central side effects and chronic headache. Common denominator may be the psychological effect – the ability of all of these drugs to relieve pain instantaneously – and this effect leads to chronic intake (see Isler, this volume). But in addition, they may have similar pharmacological effects which are the basis of their side effects in chronic abuse: effects on vascular smooth muscles, effects on prostaglandins in the vessel walls, and effects mediated by the autonomic nervous system regulating the vasculature. These effects could be regarded as causes of drug-induced headache.

Summary

Chronic daily headache was not only induced by ergotamine, as has been described already, but also by chronically ingested DHE. The daily "dosage at risk" for ergotamine and DHE is between 3 and 4 mg. Not only drugs combined with ergot derivatives and analgesics, but also minor analgesics, such as acetaminophen and salicylic acid in the usual combination with caffeine and in combinations with each other, are able to induce daily headache. Acetaminophen and salicylic acid seem to have a critical daily dosage. If more than 1000 mg are taken daily, chronic headaches may occur. Whether chronic daily intake per se or critical single and cumulative dosages play the crucial role remains to be clarified. In contrast to barbiturates, codeine dosages do not increase with daily intake of analgesic drugs, indicating a lower abuse potential. Caffeine in combination drugs seems to play a minor role in abuse, since the median dose of 300 mg per day – corresponding to three to four cups of coffee – seems to be rather low.

References

Aellig WH (1982) Agonists and antagonists of 5-hydroxytryptamine on venomotor receptors. In: Critchley M, Friedman AP, Gorini S, Sicuteri F (eds) Advances in neurology. Raven, New York, pp 321–324
Aellig WH (1984) Investigation of the venoconstrictor effect of 8′hydroxydihydroergotamine, the main metabolite of dihydroergotamine, in man. Eur J Clin Pharmacol 26:239–242

Ala-Hurula V, Myllylä V, Hokkanen E (1982) Ergotamine abuse: results of ergotamine discontinuation, with special reference to the plasma concentrations. Cephalalgia 2:189–195

Andersson PG (1975) Ergotamine headache. Headache 15:118–121

Babayan EA, Lepakhin VK, Rudenko GM (1980) Opioid analgesics and narcotic antagonists. In: Dukes MNG (ed) Meyler's side effects of drugs. Excerpta Medica, Amsterdam, pp 102–122

Beaver WT (1981) Aspirin and acetaminophen as constituents of analgesic combinations. Arch Intern Med 141:293–300

Bruce M, Scott N, Lader M, Marks V (1986) The psychopharmacological and electrophysiological effects of single doses of caffeine in healthy human subjects. Br J Clin Pharmacol 22:81–87

Dichgans J, Diener HC, Gerber WD, Verspohl EJ, Kukiolka H, Kluck M (1984) Analgetika-induzierter Dauerkopfschmerz. Dtsch Med Wochenschr 109:369–373

Gibson T, Zaphiropoulos G, Grove J, Widdop B, Berry D (1975) Kinetics of salicylate metabolism. Br J Clin Pharmacol 2:233

Henry P, Dartigues JF, Benetier MP, Lucas J, Duplan B, Jogeix M, Orgogozo JM (1985) Ergotamine- and analgesic-induced headaches. In: Rose FC (ed) Migraine. Proc 5th Int Migraine Symp London 1984. Karger, Basel, pp 197–205

Horton BT, Peters GA (1963) Clinical manifestations of excessive use of ergotamine preparations and management of withdrawal effect: report of 52 cases. Headache 3:214–226

Isler H (1982) Migraine treatment as a cause of chronic migraine. In: Rose FC (ed) Advances in migraine research and therapy. Raven, New York, pp 159–164

Kudrow L (1982) Paradoxical effects of frequent analgesic use. In: Critchley M, Friedman AP, Gorini S, Sicuteri F (eds) Advances in neurology, vol 33. Raven, New york, 335–341

Langemark M, Olesen J (1984) Drug abuse in migraine patients. Pain 19:81–86

Laska EM, Sunshine A, Mueller F, Elvers WB, Siegel C, Rubin A (1984) Caffeine as an analgesic adjuvant. JAMA 251:1711–1718

Linblad B, Abisch E, Bergqvist D (1983) The pharmacokinetics of subcutaneous dihydroergotamine with and without dextran 70 infusion. Eur J Clin Pharmacol 24:813–818

Lippman CW (1955) Characteristic headache resulting from prolonged use of ergot derivatives. J Nerv Ment Dis 121:270–273

Mathew RJ, Wilson WH (1985) Caffeine consumption, withdrawal and cerebral blood flow, Headache 25:305–309

Mathew NT, Stubits E, Nigam MP (1982) Transformation of episodic migraine into daily chronic headache: analysis of factors. Headache 22:66–68

Maurer G, Frick W (1984) Elucidation of the structure and receptor binding studies of the major primary metabolite of dihydroergotamine in man. Eur J Clin Pharmacol 26:463–470

Meadows BJ (1984) Codeine combinations in clinical practise. Curr Ther Res 35:501–510

Müller-Schweinitzer E, Fanchamps A (1982) Effects on arterial receptors of ergot derivatives used in migraine. In: Critchley M, Friedman AP, Gorini S, Sicuteri F (eds) Advances in neurology. Raven, New York, pp 343–356

Pincomb GA, Lovallo WR, Passay RB, Whitsett TL, Silverstein SM, Wilson MF (1985) Effects of caffeine on vascular resistance, cardiac output and myocardial contractility in young men. Am J Cardiol 56:119–122

Rapoport A, Weeks R, Sheftell F et al. (1985) Analgesic rebound headache: theoretical and practical implications. In: Olesen J, Tfelt-Hansen P, Jensen K (eds) Headache 1985. Proceedings of the second international headache congress. Jensen, Copenhagen, pp 448–449

Rowsell AR, Neylan C, Wilkinson M (1973) Ergotamine induced headaches in migrainous patients. Headache 13:65–67

Saper JR (1983) Drug abuse among headache patients. In: Saper JR (ed) Headache disorders: current concepts and treatment strategies. Wright, Boston, pp 263–278

Saxena PR (1982) Agonists and antagonists of vascular receptors. In: Critchley M, Friedman AP, Gorini S, Sicuteri F (eds) Advances in neurology. Raven, New York, pp 309–314

Svihovec J (1980) Anti-inflammatory analgesics and drugs used in gout. In: Dukes MNG (ed) Meyler's side effects of drugs. Excerpta Medica, Amsterdam, pp 141–164

Tfelt-Hansen P (1986) The effect of ergotamine on the arterial system in man. Acta Pharmacol Toxicol 59: [Suppl 3] 7–29

Tfelt-Hansen P, Eickhoff JH, Olesen J (1982) Duration of the biological effect of ergotamine tartrate. In: Critchley M, Friedman AP, Gorini S, Sicuteri F (eds) Advances in neurology. Raven, New York, pp 315–319

Wainscott G, Volans G, Wilkinson M (1974) Ergotamine induced headaches. Br Med J ii:724

Wilkinson M (1983) Treatment of the acute migraine attack – current status. Cephalalgia 3:61–67

Woodbury DM, Fingl E (1975) Analgesic-antipyretics, anti-inflammatory agents, and drugs employed in the therapy of gout. In: Goodman LS, Gilman A (eds) The pharmacological basis of therapeutics. Macmillan, New York, pp 325–358

Woodcock BG, Loh W, Habedank W-D, Rietbrock N (1982) Dihydrotoxine kinetics in healthy men after intravenous and oral administration. Clin Pharmacol Ther 32:622–627

What Kind of Drugs Are Taken
by Patients with Primary Headaches?

V. Pfaffenrath[1] and U. Niederberger[2]

The daily or almost daily intake of monoanalgesics, analgesic and ergotamine combinations, or opioids may, in patients with primary headaches, cause a continuous headache, which is defined as "analgesic-induced rebound headache" (Andersson 1975; Hokkanen et al. 1978; Tfelt-Hausen and Krabbe 1981). This drug-induced headache occurs predominantly in patients suffering from migraine (Andersson 1975; Mathew et al. 1982; Wilkinson 1983) tension headache (Rapoport 1984; Ziegler 1985), or combination headache (which is a combination of migraine and tension headache) (Mathew 1981; Saper 1982; Pfaffenrath et al. 1986) and manifests itself, mainly at alternating sides and as a daily, partly throbbing, partly dull headache (Kudrow 1982; Rapoport 1984) with accompanying minor vegetative and visual symptoms. The analgesic-induced headache resembles the basic primary headache, and its differentiation from the latter causes major problems, both for the affected patient and the physician. It is maintained by a sometimes almost careless use of analgesics, by the patients fear of the next attack and finally by his addiction to the barbiturates and opioids contained in the compound preparations (Wörz 1983; Dichgans et al. 1984; Rapoport 1984). After a period of habituation due to the psychotropic effects of barbiturates and opioids, a psychophysical dependence results, which might be enhanced in individual cases by an abuse of tranquilizers.

The patients attitude toward drugs is also influenced by the drug experience of headache sufferers in his close environment (Tfelt-Hansen 1985). Usually, the drug dosage necessary to reduce the pain is increased over months and years (Rapoport 1984). The attempt to treat the disease by means of potent headache prophylactics has to fail as long as analgesics are taken daily. This explains the long course of the headache disease and the final self-administration of drugs by the patient without any medical control. The effort of medically informed patients to reduce their analgesic intake by themselves or even to stop it fails for the following reasons:

- The withdrawal headache caused by the abrupt discontinuation of the medication, which may last from 3 days to 3 weeks (Dichgans et al. 1984; Rapoport 1984), resembles the basic headache syndrome and results in a rapid resumption of self-administration
- The successful treatment of the analgesic-induced headache requires the immediate discontinuation of all analgesics. A dose reduction alone will not influence the symptoms

[1] Leopoldstr. 59/II, 8000 München 40, Federal Republic of Germany
[2] Department of Neuropsychology, Universität Tübingen, Gartenstr. 29, 7400 Tübingen, Federal Republic of Germany

Drug-Induced Headache
Ed. by H.-C. Diener and M. Wilkinson
© Springer-Verlag Berlin Heidelberg 1988

– After regression of the withdrawal headache, the primary headache persists unchanged. If adequate prophylaxis is not introduced concomitantly, self-administration will soon recommence (Kudrow 1982)

Thus, the successful treatment of a patient with an analgesic-induced headache depends on the knowledge of the mechanisms which induce and maintain the pain and moreover requires that the patient has full medical information. Whether the analgesic withdrawal is carried out on an out- or inpatient basis depends on the therapeutist's experience.

In summary, the literature (Kudrow 1982; Wörz 1983; Dichgans et al. 1984) provides sufficient information about the diagnosis and treatment of analgesic-induced headache. So far, however, these findings are not based on extensive case material. Therefore, the drug-taking behavior of a total of 1435 headache patients is described below.

Material and Methods

Material

This study comprises 1435 outpatients who consulted the Department of Neurology, Klinikum Großhadern, University of Munich, between 1981 and 1985. The primary headaches were diagnosed according to the criteria of the WFN Research Group of Migraine and Headache and the Ad Hoc Committee on Classification of Headache (1962).

The data were collected by means of a standardized questionnaire at the patient's first presentation. Each patient was submitted to careful neurologic examinations and routine laboratory parameters were assessed. Some clinical parameters and the drug consumption of the individual diagnostic groups (migraine, tension headache, and combination headache) are reviewed.

Statistical Evaluation

The statistical evaluation was performed descriptively.

Results

Patients

The total group comprised 1435 outpatients (1022 female, 413 male) aged between 8 and 82 years ($\bar{X} = 32.9$ years). The age and sex distribution is shown in Table 1. Of the patients 42.9% suffered from migraine, 15.2% from tension headache and 29.4% from combination headache. Cluster headache (Kudrow 1979) was diagnosed in 3.6%. As has been reported in the literature, migraine and com-

Table 1. Age and sex distribution in 1435 patients with primary headaches

Diagnosis	Sex		(n)	(%)	Age	
	Male	Female			Mean	Range
Migraine	154	461	615	42.9	36.1	8–69
Tension headache	98	120	218	15.2	41.6	13–81
Combination headache	85	336	421	29.4	40.6	14–82
Cluster headache	36	16	52	3.6	42.4	17–79
Other head and face pains	40	89	129	9.0	44.3	16–79
Total	413	1022	1435	100.0	39.2	8–82

bination headache were mostly seen in females and cluster headache in males. There was only a slightly higher frequency of tension headache in women.

The group suffering from "other head and facial pains" ($n=129$) included 61 patients (4.3%) with cervicogenic headache (17), 29 patients (2%) with trigeminal neuralgia, 13 patients (0.9%) with chronic paroxysmal hemicrania (18), nine cases (0.6%) with psychogenic headache and atypical face pain and two patients (0.2%) with coital headache (Lundberg and Osterman 1974). The small number of patients with trigeminal neuralgia is explained by the fact that these cases are usually referred to our Neurosurgical Outpatient Department for facial pain.

Analgesic Drugs

Migraine

The 615 migraine patients (461 female, 154 male) aged between 8 and 69 years ($\bar{X}=36.1$ years) suffered mostly from common migraine (81.1%), followed by those with a complicated (8.8%) and classical migraine (5.2%). "Classical migraine" was defined as a headache succeeding a typical visual aura with or without other focal-neurological symptoms.

Headaches, which were either preceded by a focal-neurological deficit (without a visual aura), or which accompanied the headache or even outlasted it, were referred to as "complicated migraine." A total of 3.3% had menstrual migraine (Welch et al. 1984), 1.5% had cluster migraine (Sjaastad 1986), a combination of cluster and migraine symptoms. Apart from cluster migraine, there was a clear prevalence of women in all groups (Table 2).

Of the 615 migraine patients, about 32% had suffered from attacks since childhood, and 57.4% had a family history of migraine. Both groups showed a comparable sex distribution (Table 3). Altogether, the average migraine duration was 15.5 years ($\tilde{X}=12.4$, SD$=10.9$), with women suffering longer than men. The frequency of attacks was reported to be 4.7 per month ($\tilde{X}=4.0$, SD$=3.83$), whereas the length of an attack was said to be 1.7 days ($\tilde{X}=2.0$, SD$=0.97$)

Table 2. Age and sex distribution in 615 migraine patients

Diagnosis	Sex		(n)	(%)	Age	
	Male	Female			Mean	Range
Common migraine	124	375	499	81.1	36.1	8–69
Classical migraine	9	23	32	5.2	38.6	13–63
Complicated migraine	17	38	55	8.8	28.5	14–55
Menstrual migraine		20	20	3.3	35.8	18–47
Cluster migraine	4	5	9	1.5	36.3	20–63
Total	154	461	615	100.0	36.1	8–69

Table 3. Family history of headaches and headaches in childhood in 615 migraine patients

Sex	Headaches in childhood						Family history of headache					
	Yes		No		Missing data		Yes		No		Missing data	
	(n)	(%)	(n)	(%)	(n)	(%)	(n)	(%)	(n)	(%)	(n)	(%)
Female	141	30.6	297	64.4	23	5.0	264	57.3	149	32.3	48	10.4
Male	55	35.7	96	62.3	3	1.9	89	57.8	58	37.7	7	4.5
Total	196	31.9	393	63.9	26	4.2	353	57.4	207	33.7	55	8.9

Table 4. Frequency and duration of the single migraine attack and duration of the disease in 615 migraine patients

Statistics	Duration of the disease (years)			Attack frequency per month			Attack duration in days		
	Female	Male	Total	Female	Male	Total	Female	Male	Total
Mean	15.8	14.5	15.5	4.5	5.1	4.7	1.8	1.4	1.7
$\tilde{x}$	13.1	11.7	12.4	4.0	4.0	4.0	2.0	1.0	2.0
SD	10.8	11.4	10.9	3.78	3.96	3.38	0.97	0.8	0.97

(Table 4). Tables 5 and 6 subdivide the duration and frequency of the individual attacks and show that in 68.9% of the migraine patients the attacks lasted about 1–2 days and in about 60% they were experienced two to six times per month. On the whole, it may be assumed that these migraine sufferers represent a negative selection which seems to be predisposed to drug abuse because of the long persistence of the disease and the high rate of attacks.

Table 7 reflects the number of analgesic intakes per month by the migraine group. Ergotamine combinations prevailed (37.3%), followed by analgesic combinations (36.8%) and monosubstance analgesics (12.9%). A series of other pain killers (e.g., spasmolytics) was used by 51 (8.3%) patients. Daily, or almost daily, ergotamine combinations were consumed by 9%, analgesic combinations by

Table 5. Duration of the single migraine attack in 615 migraine patients

Duration	Sex		(n)	(%)
	Female	Male		
1–6 h	24	12	36	5.9
7–18 h	40	18	58	9.4
1 day	126	68	194	31.5
2 days	188	42	230	37.4
3 days	46	7	53	8.6
4 days	19	3	22	3.6
5 days	4	1	5	0.8
6 days	1	0	1	0.2
Missing data	13	3	16	2.6
Total	461	154	615	100.0

Table 6. Frequency of attacks per month in 615 migraine patients

Frequency per month	Male		Female		Total	
	(n = 154)	(%)	(n = 461)	(%)	(n = 615)	(%)
< 1	9	5.8	19	4.1	28	4.6
1	11	7.1	57	12.4	68	11.1
2	18	11.7	68	14.8	86	14.0
3	22	14.3	66	14.3	88	14.3
4	25	16.2	84	18.2	109	17.7
5	8	5.2	44	9.5	52	8.5
6	17	11.0	16	3.5	33	5.4
7–10	27	17.5	58	12.6	85	13.8
11–24	10	6.5	33	7.3	43	7.1
Missing data	7	4.6	16	3.5	23	3.7

Table 7. Intake of mixed ergot and analgesic compounds and simple analgesics per month in 615 migraine patients

Frequency per month	Mixed ergot preparations[a]			Mixed analgesics[a]			Analgesics[a]		
	(n)	(%)[b]	(%)[c]	(n)	(%)[a]	(%)[e]	(n)	(%)[f]	(%)[g]
1– 10	132	57.6	21.5	136	60.2	22.2	59	74.7	9.6
11– 20	42	18.3	6.8	44	19.5	7.2	9	11.4	1.5
21– 30	17	7.5	2.8	13	5.8	2.1	5	6.3	0.8
31– 60	27	11.8	4.4	15	6.6	2.4	5	6.3	0.8
61–150	11	4.8	1.8	13	5.8	2.1	1	1.3	0.2
151–300	–	–	–	5	2.2	0.8	–	–	–
Total	229	100.0	37.3	226	100.0	36.8	79	100.0	12.9

[a] More than one quotation possible.　　　　[e] $n = 615 \simeq 100\%$.
[b] $n = 229 \simeq 100\%$.　　　　[f] $n = 79 \simeq 100\%$.
[c] $n = 615 \simeq 100\%$.　　　　[g] $n = 615 \simeq 100\%$.
[d] $n = 226 \simeq 100\%$.

Table 8. Intake of pain killers in 615 migraine patients

Drugs	One pain killer		>One pain killer[b]	
	(n)	(%)[a]	(n)	(%)[a]
Mixed ergots	98	15.9	131	21.3
Mixed analgesics	85	13.8	141	22.9
Analgesics	36	5.9	43	7.0
Others	17	2.8	34	6.2
Total	236	38.4	183	29.8

[a] $n = 615 \cong 100\%$.
[b] More than one quotation possible.

6.6% and monoanalgesics by 1.8%. 38.4% of all migraine patients took only one analgesic drug, while nearly 29.8% consumed different substances (up to five) concomitantly (Table 8).

The composition of the different analgesic drugs is shown in Tables 9–11. With regard to analgesic and ergotamine combinations, there is evidence that substances with a known potential for drug dependence, like barbiturates and codeine, were taken more often. The ergotamine doses administered in combination with one or two monoanalgesics are sufficient to induce chronic headaches. While according to the present status of attack treatment (Wilkinson 1983), an antiemetic drug combined with a simple analgesic, such as acetylicsalicylic acid or paracetamol, should be used in the first instance and ergotamine preparations only afterwards, there was no evidence for such an approach in the migraine group studied.

Tension Headache

A total of 218 patients (15.2%) including 120 women and 98 men with a mean age of 41.6 years (13–81 years) suffered from tension headache. In contrast to those with a mere migraine, only 26.6% of these cases had a family history of headache. Only 7.3% reported an onset during childhood (Table 12). According to the patients descriptions, most headaches – those occurring in childhood as well as the familial ones – did rather resemble migraine.

Table 13 lists some parameters concerning the duration of the disease. According to these data, the tension headache lasted 10 years on average ($\tilde{X} = 6.7$, SD = 9.4). Daily headaches with a mean length of 11 h ($\tilde{X} = 9.1$, SD = 9.1) had been present for 5.7 years ($\tilde{X} = 3.0$, SD = 7.1).

As expected, the patients with tension headache preferred analgesic combinations (31.9%), followed by ergotamine combinations (14.5%) and analgesic monopreparations (13.8%). The lack of effect of ergotamine on tension headache becomes apparent here. There was a daily or almost daily abuse of monoanalgesics in 6.4%, of ergotamine combinations in 7.9%, and of analgesic combinations in 18.5% of cases (Table 14).

Table 9. Mixed ergot compounds[a] in 615 migraine patients

Trade name	(n)	(%)[b]	Compound[c]	(mg)
Cafergot PB	72	11.7	Ergotamine tartrate	1
			Butalbital	50
			Belladonna Alkaloids	0.125
			Caffeine	100
Ergo-Lonarid	46	7.5	Dihydroergotamine	0.5
			Paracetamol	400
			Codeine	10
			Caffeine	100
Ergo-Sanol	44	7.2	Ergotamine tartrate	0.25
			Caffeine	60
			Ethencamid	100
			Vitamine B_1	5
Avamigran	42	6.8	Ergotamine tartrate	0.75
			Propyphenazone	200
			Camylofin	25
			Caffeine	80
			Mecloxamine	20
Optalidon spezial	25	4.1	Dihydroergotamine	0.5
			Propyphenazone	125
			Butalbital	50
			Caffeine	40
Migräne-Dolviran	19	3.1	Ergotamine tartrate	0.75
			Acetylicsalicylic acid	400
			Codeine	9.6
			Caffeine	50
Migrexa	8	1.3	Ergotamine tartrate	1
			Pentobarbital	25
			Caffeine	50
Ergo-Kranit	7	1.1	Ergotamine tartrate	0.75
			Propyphenazone	150
			Paracetamol	200
			Phenobarbital	30
			Caffeine	85

[a] From the drugs mentioned, 102 were administered as tablets, nine as dragees and 142 as suppositories.
[b] $n = 615 \cong 100\%$.
[c] Average dosage of tablets.

A total of 27.2% of the patients took only a single drug, which was an ergotamine combination in 14.2% and an analgesic combination in 6.4% of the cases. A further 20.6% consumed drugs of different substance groups, with ergotamine combinations predominating in 17.4% of the patients, followed by monoanalgesics in 8.7% and analgesic combinations in 7.8% (Table 15). The comparison of the preparations preferred by the tension headache patients (Tables 16–18) with those favored by the migraine patients revealed no major difference. Here again codeine- and barbiturate-containing preparations took the lead.

Table 10. Mixed analgesics in 615 migraine patients[a]

Trade name	(n)	(%)[b]	Compounds[c]	(mg)
Thomapyrin	59	9.6	Acetylicsalicylic acid Paracetamol Caffeine	250 200 50
Migräne-Kranit	35	5.7	Paracetamol Propyphenazone Phenobarbital Caffeine	200 150 30 85
Optalidon	34	5.5	Propyphenazone Butalbital Caffeine	125 50 25
Spasmo-Cibalgin	22	3.6	Propyphenazone Codeine	220 20
Gelonida	20	3.3	Acetylicsalicylic acid Paracetamol Codeine	250 250 10
Spalt	13	2.1	Phenazone salicylate Salicylamide Caffeine	225 225 50
Vivimed	15	2.4	Paracetamol Propyphenazone Caffeine Vitamin B_1	150 155 50 5
Dolviran	8	1.3	Acetylicsalicylic acid Codeine Caffeine	400 9.6 50
Silentan	7	1.1	Acetylicsalicylic acid Diazepame	400 2
Others	37	6.3	Other compounds, containing analgesics, barbiturates, and codeine	

[a] From the drugs mentioned, 173 were administered as tablets, five as dragees and 53 as suppositories.
[b] $n = 615 \simeq 100\%$.
[c] Average dosage in tablets and dragees.

Table 11. Simple analgesics in 615 migraine patients[a]

Trade name[b]	(n)	(%)[c]	Compound	(mg)
Aspirin	40	6.5	Acetylicsalicylic acid	500
Novalgin	20	3.3	Metamizole	500
Ben-u-ron	7	1.1	Paracetamol	500
Others	2	0.4	–	–

[a] All drugs given as tablets.
[b] More than one quotation possible.
[c] $n = 615 \simeq 100\%$.

Table 12. Family history of headaches and headaches in childhood in 218 tension headache patients

Sex	Headaches in childhood						Family history of headache					
	Yes		No		Missing data		Yes		No		Missing data	
	(n)	$(\%)$	(n)	$(\%)$	(n)	$(\%)$	(n)	$(\%)$	(n)	$(\%)$	(n)	$(\%)$
Female	8	6.7	106	88.3	6	5.0	33	27.5	62	51.7	25	20.8
Male	8	8.2	80	81.6	10	10.2	25	25.5	51	52.0	22	22.4
Total	16	7.3	186	85.4	16	7.3	58	26.6	113	51.8	47	21.6

Table 13. Duration of the disease and duration per day in 218 tension headache patients

Statistics	Female	Male	Total
Duration (years)			
$\bar{X}$	9.4	10.6	10.0
$\tilde{X}$	6.4	7.5	6.7
SD	8.5	10.4	9.4
Duration of daily headaches (years)			
$\bar{X}$	5.6	5.8	5.7
$\tilde{X}$	3.0	3.0	3.0
SD	7.0	7.2	7.1
Duration of tension headaches (h per day)			
$\bar{X}$	9.7	12.6	11.0
$\tilde{X}$	10.0	8.9	9.1
SD	6.5	16.2	9.1

Table 14. Intake of mixed ergot and analgesics compounds and simple analgesics per month in 218 tension headache patients

Frequency per months	Mixed ergot preparations			Mixed analgesics			Analgesics		
	(n)	$(\%)^a$	$(\%)^b$	(n)	$(\%)^c$	$(\%)^d$	(n)	$(\%)^e$	$(\%)^f$
1– 10	9	29.0	4.3	24	34.9	11.1	13	43.3	6.0
11– 20	5	16.1	2.3	5	7.2	2.3	3	10.0	1.4
21– 30	5	16.1	2.3	9	13.0	4.1	4	16.3	1.8
31– 60	6	19.3	2.8	8	11.6	3.8	5	16.7	2.3
61–150	6	19.4	2.8	15	21.7	6.9	3	10.0	1.4
151–300	–	–	–	8	11.6	3.7	2	6.6	0.9
Total	31	100.0	14.5	69	100.0	31.9	30	100.0	13.8

[a] $n = \ 31 \simeq 100\%$.
[b] $n = 218 \simeq 100\%$.
[c] $n = \ 69 \simeq 100\%$.
[d] $n = 218 \simeq 100\%$.
[e] $n = \ 30 \simeq 100\%$.
[f] $n = 218 \simeq 100\%$.

Table 15. Intake of pain killers in 218 tension headache patients

Drugs	One pain killer		>One pain killer[b]	
	(n)	$(\%)^a$	(n)	$(\%)^a$
Mixed ergots	31	14.2	38	17.4
Mixed analgesics	14	6.4	17	7.8
Analgesics	11	5.1	19	8.7
Others	4	1.5	10	4.7
Total	60	27.2	45	20.6

[a] $n = 218 \simeq 100\%$.
[b] More than one quotation possible.

Table 16. Mixed analgesics in 218 tension headache patients[a]

Trade name[b]	(n)	(%)[c]	Compounds[d]	(mg)
Thomapyrin	26	11.9	Acetylicsalicylic acid	250
			Paracetamol	200
			Caffeine	50
Optalidon	13	6.0	Propyphenazone	125
			Butalbital	50
			Caffeine	25
Silentan	9	4.1	Acetylicsalicylic acid	400
			Diazepame	2
Gelonida	7	3.2	Acetylicsalicylic acid	250
			Paracetamol	250
			Codeine	90
Vivimed	7	3.2	Paracetamol	150
			Propyphenazone	155
			Caffeine	50
			Vitamin B_1	5
Migräne-Kranit	6	2.8	Paracetamol	200
			Propyphenazone	150
			Phenobarbital	30
			Caffeine	85
Others	30	14.0		

[a] From the drugs mentioned, 62 were administered as tablets, six as dragees and four as suppositories.
[b] $n = 218 \cong 100\%$.
[c] More than one quotation possible.
[d] Average dosage in tablets and dragees.

Combination Headache

Of the 421 Patients (336 female, 85 male) with a combination headache, aged between 14 and 82 years ($\bar{X} = 40.6$ years), 34.9% complained of pains since their childhood. There was a familial history of headaches in 57.4% of the cases. On the whole, the data corresponded with those of the migraine patients (Table 19). Altogether, the mean duration of the migraine disease was 18.5 years ($\tilde{X} = 15.8$, SD $= 12.9$). The frequency of attacks amounted to 4.3 per month ($\tilde{X} = 4.0$, SD $= 3.1$), whereas the average length of an attack was 1.8 days ($\tilde{X} = 1.9$, SD $= 1.0$) (Table 20).

Taken together, the tension headache had been part of the combination headache for 12.9 years ($\tilde{X} = 10.0$, SD $= 10.0$) and daily headaches commenced 8.5 years ago ($\tilde{X} = 5.0$, SD $= 8.9$). On average, the tension headache lasted 11.3 h ($\tilde{X} = 11.6$, SD $= 7.6$) per day (Table 21).

As expected, drugs were abused above all by the group with combination headache. Analgesic combinations were taken in 45.1%, 23.6% of which were used daily or almost daily. They were succeeded by a 41.1% intake of ergotamine combinations, 19.9% of which were used daily to almost daily. Monoanalgesics

Table 17. Mixed ergots in 218 tension headache patients[a]

Trade name[b]	(n)	(%)[c]	Compound[d]	(mg)
Ergo-Lonarid	14	6.4	Dihydroergotamine	0.5
			Paracetamol	400
			Codeine	10
			Caffeine	100
Optalidon spezial	5	2.3	Dihydroergotamine	0.5
			Propyphenazone	125
			Butalbital	50
			Caffeine	40
Ergo-Sanol	4	1.8	Ergotamine tartrate	0.25
			Caffeine	60
			Ethencamid	100
			Vitamine B_1	5
Avamigran	4	1.8	Ergotamine tartrate	0.75
			Propyphenazone	200
			Camylofin	25
			Caffeine	80
			Mecloxamine	20
Cafergot PB	2	0.9	Ergotamine tartrate	1
			Butalbital	50
			Belladonna alkaloids	0.125
			Caffeine	100
Migrexa	1	0.5	Ergotamine tartrate	1
			Pentobarbital	25
			Caffeine	50
Celetil	1	0.5	Ergotamine tartrate	1
			Caffeine	100

[a] From the drugs mentioned, 20 were administered as tablets, one as a dragee, and ten as suppositories.
[b] More than one quotation possible.
[c] $n = 218 \cong 100\%$.
[d] Average dosage of tablets.

Table 18. Simple analgesics in 218 tension headache patients[a]

Trade name[b]	(n)	(%)[c]	Compound	(mg)
Aspirin	17	7.8	Acetylicsalicylic acid	500
Novalgin	5	2.3	Metamizole	500
Ben-u-ron	1	0.5	Paracetamol	500

[a] All drugs given as tablets.
[b] More than one quotation possible.
[c] $n = 218 \cong 100\%$.

Table 19. Headaches in childhood and family history of headaches in 421 patients with combination headache

Sex	Headaches in childhood						Family history of headache					
	Yes		No		Missing data		Yes		No		Missing data	
	(n)	(%)	(n)	(%)	(n)	(%)	(n)	(%)	(n)	(%)	(n)	(%)
Female	118	35.1	206	61.3	12	3.6	190	56.6	116	34.5	30	8.9
Male	29	34.1	54	63.5	2	2.4	35	41.2	40	47.1	10	11.8
Total	147	34.9	260	61.8	14	3.3	225	57.4	156	33.7	40	8.9

Table 20. Migraine frequency and duration of the disease in 421 patients with combination headache

	Duration of the disease (years)			Attack frequency per month			Attack duration (days)		
	Female	Male	Total	Female	Male	Total	Female	Male	Total
$\bar{X}$	18.4	18.7	18.5	4.1	4.9	4.3	1.8	1.4	1.8
$\tilde{X}$	16.2	14.7	15.8	4.0	4.0	4.0	2.0	1.0	1.9
SD	12.2	12.0	12.9	3.0	3.2	3.1	1.0	0.6	1.0

Table 21. Duration of tension headache and duration of the disease in 421 patients with combination headache

Statistics	Female	Male	Total
Duration of tension headache (years)			
$\bar{X}$	13.0	12.7	12.9
$\tilde{X}$	10.0	10.0	10.0
SD	9.9	10.5	10.0
Duration of daily headaches (years)			
$\bar{X}$	8.6	7.7	8.5
$\tilde{X}$	5.0	5.0	5.0
SD	8.7	9.7	8.9
Duration of tension headache (h per day)			
$\bar{X}$	11.4	11.1	11.3
$\tilde{X}$	9.5	11.8	11.6
SD	7.8	6.9	7.6

Table 22. Intake of mixed ergots and analgesics compounds and simple analgesics per month in 421 patients with combination headache

Frequency per month	Mixed ergot preparations			Mixed analgesics			Analgesics		
	(n)	$(\%)^a$	$(\%)^b$	(n)	$(\%)^c$	$(\%)^d$	(n)	$(\%)^e$	$(\%)^f$
1– 10	49	28.5	11.9	68	36.0	16.3	29	58.0	6.9
11– 20	39	22.7	9.3	22	11.6	5.2	9	18.0	2.1
21– 30	30	17.4	7.1	23	12.2	5.5	2	18.0	2.1
31– 60	27	15.7	6.4	31	16.4	7.4	3	6.0	0.7
61–150	21	12.2	5.0	31	16.4	7.4	3	6.0	0.7
151–300	6	3.5	1.4	14	7.4	3.3	4	8.0	1.0
Total	172	100.0	41.1	189	100.0	45.1	50	100.0	13.5

[a] $n = 172 \cong 100\%$.
[b] $n = 421 \cong 100\%$.
[c] $n = 189 \cong 100\%$.
[d] $n = 421 \cong 100\%$.
[e] $n = 50 \cong 100\%$.
[f] $n = 421 \cong 100\%$.

Table 23. Intake of pain killers in 421 patients with combination headache

	One pain killer		>One pain killer[b]	
	(n)	$(\%)^a$	(n)	$(\%)^a$
Mixed ergots	73	17.3	99	23.5
Mixed analgesics	65	15.4	124	29.5
Analgesics	13	3.1	37	8.8
Others	8	2.0	22	5.3
Total	159	37.8	144	34.2

[a] $n = 415 \cong 100\%$.
[b] More than one quotation possible.

Table 24. Mixed ergot preparatories in 421 patients with combination headache[a]

Trade name[b]	(n)	(%)[c]	Compound[d]	(mg)
Ergo-Lonarid	51	12.1	Dihydroergotamine	0.5
			Paracetamol	400
			Codeine	10
			Caffeine	100
Cafergot PB	36	8.6	Ergotamine tartrate	1
			Butalbital	50
			Belladonna alkaloids	0.125
			Caffeine	100
Optalidon spezial	35	8.3	Dihydroergotamine	0.5
			Propyphenazone	125
			Butalbital	50
			Caffeine	40
Avamigran	26	6.2	Ergotamine tartrate	0.75
			Propyphenazone	200
			Camylofin	25
			Caffeine	80
			Mecloxamine	20
Ergo-Sanol	23	5.5	Ergotamine tartrate	0.25
			Caffeine	60
			Ethencamid	100
			Vitamin B_1	5
Migrexa	10	2.4	Ergotamine tartrate	1
			Pentobarbital	25
			Caffeine	50
Ergo-Kranit	9	2.1	Ergotamine tartrate	0.75
			Propyphenazone	150
			Paracetamol	200
			Phenobarbital	30
			Caffeine	85
Migräne-Dolviran	2	0.5	Ergotamine tartrate	0.75
			Acetylicsalicylic acid	400
			Codeine	9.6
			Caffeine	50
Celetil	2	0.5	Ergotamine tartrate	1
			Caffeine	100
Praecimal	1	0.2	Ergotamine tartrate	0.75
			Caffeine	
Others	1	0.2	–	–

[a] The drug mentioned were administered in 104 patients as tablets, in eight as dragees, and in 75 as suppositories.
[b] More than one quotation possible.
[c] $n = 421 \cong 100\%$.
[d] Average dosage of tablets.

Table 25. Mixed analgesics in 421 patients with combination headache[a]

Trade name[b]	(*n*)	(%)[c]	Compound[d]	(mg)
Thomapyrin	53	12.6	Acetylicsalicylic acid Paracetamol Caffeine	250 200 50
Optalidon	27	6.4	Propyphenazone Butalbital Caffeine	125 50 25
Migräne-Kranit	23	5.5	Paracetamol Propyphenazone Phenobarbital Caffeine	200 150 30 85
Silentan	19	4.5	Acetylicsalicylic acid Diazepame	400 2
Spasmo-Cibalgin	17	4.0	Propyphenazone Codeine	220 20
Vivimed	17	4.0	Paracetamol Propyphenazone Caffeine Vitamine B_1	150 155 50 5
Spalt	15	3.6	Phenazone salicylate Salicylamide Caffeine	225 225 50
Neosal	10	2.4	Metamizole Caffeine Isometheptene	400 55 52.3
Dolviran	8	1.9	Acetylicsalicylic acid Codeine Caffeine	400 9.6 50
Gelonida	7	1.7	Acetylicsalicylic acid Paracetamol Codeine	250 250 90
Dolomo	5	1.2	Acetylicsalicylic acid Paracetamol Caffeine	250 250 50
Eumed	5	1.2	Acetylicsalicylic acid Ethencamid Caffeine	400 100 50
Migränex	2	0.5	Phenyldimethylpyrazolone Caffeine	400
Others	16	3.6		

[a] The drugs mentioned were administered in 144 patients as tablets, in four as dagrees and in 23 as suppositories.
[b] More than one quotation possible.
[c] $n = 421 \cong 100\%$.
[d] Average dosage in tablets and dragees.

Table 26. Simple analgesics in 421 patients with combination headache[a]

Trade name[b]	(n)	(%)[c]	Compound	(mg)
Aspirin	20	4.8	Acetylicsalicylic acid	500
Novalgin	13	3.1	Metamizole	500
Togal	5	1.2	Acetylicsalicylic acid	250
Ben-u-ron	3	0.7	Paracetamol	500
Others	2	0.4	–	–

[a] All drugs given in tablets.
[b] More than one quotation possible.
[c] $n = 421 \cong 100\%$.

were consumed by 13.5%, with 4.5% using them more or less regularly (Table 22).

A single drug was taken by 37.8% of the patients. In this group 17.3% preferred an ergotamine combination, 15.4% an analgesic combination and 3.1% analgesics alone. There was a concurrent intake of more than one drug in 34.2% of the patients. Here again, the analgesic combinations dominated with 29.5%, followed by ergotamine combinations with 23.5%, and simple analgesics with 8.8% (Table 23). As to the substances preferred, the Tables 24–26 show no significant differences between the patients with combination headache and those with migraine or tension headache.

Headache Prophylactics

Considering the prophylactics supplied, the discrepancy between the current status of headache treatment (Louis et al. 1982; Weerasuriya 1982; Diamond and Scheubaum 1983) and the actual medication in the patient group becomes even more significant. Table 27 demonstrates our therapeutic approach to the prophylaxis of the various forms of headache. At their first attendance, only 27 patients (4.4%) used a prophylactic, with nine of them (1.5%) each taking lisuride or dihydroergotamine, seven (1.1%) pizotifen and two (0.3%) clonidine. Only four (0.7%) patients had received a beta-blocker (propranolol) and this was in an insufficient dosage.

In the case of migraine, beta-blockers and flunarizine or a combination of both substances predominated in our treatment. A total of 35.1% of the migraine patients with fewer than two attacks per month needed only single attack medication.

Only two (0.9%) of the 218 patients with tension headache were initially given amitriptyline (each at a maximum dosage of 25 mg per day), five others (2.4%) dihydroergotamine, one each (0.5%) clonidine or propranolol. A benzodiazepeine preparation was used almost daily in three patients (1.4%).

A total of 78.9% of our tension headache group were treated with a tricyclic antidepressive – either amitriptyline or amitriptyline-N-oxide (Pfaffenrath et al. 1986) (Table 27).

In the 421 patients suffering from combination headache, three patients (0.7%) had each been earlier treated with clonidine and pizotifen, one (0.2%) with both methysergide and lisuride. Six (1.3%) had had dihydroergotamine, three

Table 27. Prophylactic medication in 1435 patients with primary headache

Medication	All headache patients		Migraine		Tension headache		Combination headache	
	(*n*)	(%)	(*n*)	(%)	(*n*)	(%)	(*n*)	(%)
β-Blocker	249	17.4	231	37.6	1	0.5	11	2.6
Flunarizine	75	5.2	61	9.9			17	2.9
Tricyclic antidepressives	246	17.1	4	0.7	172	78.9	52	12.4
β-Blocker + flunarizine	57	4.0	52	8.5			3	0.2
β-Blocker + tricyclic antidepressives	195	13.6	26	4.2			161	38.2
Flunarizine + tricyclic antidepressives	73	5.1	9	1.6			64	15.7
β-Blocker + flunarizine + tricyclic antidepressives	107	7.5	16	2.6	1	0.5	90	21.4
Other medication	433	30.2	216	35.1	44	20.1	28	6.7
Total	1435	100.0	615	100.0	218	100.0	421	100.0

(0.6%) opioids and tranquilizers. Only two (0.5%) had had propranolol, flunarizine, or amitriptyline. In this group we prescribed a beta-blocker (metoprolol, propranolol) combined with a tricyclic antidepressive in 38.2% of the cases. Flunarizine was given additively in 21.4% of the patients (Table 27).

Discussion

Every experienced headache therapeutist is familiar with the problem of drug abuse. Nevertheless, the findings presented above once again emphasize the extent of drug intake in a group of 1435 patients and lead to the following conclusions:

- Drug abuse develops over several years. Presumably, many of these patients practice self-medication without medical control. Neither patients nor physicians seem to be sufficiently informed about the mechanism of pain induction.
- Modern concepts on how the attacks should be routinely treated have not yet been adopted. This alone might explain the frequent administration of ergotamine and analgesic combinations despite their high potential for abuse and dependence.
- Only an extremely small percentage of the individual groups diagnosed received adequate prophylactic therapy. This refers to the antidepressives used in the treatment of tension headache as well as to the beta-blockers and flunarizine used in migraine prophylaxis.
- The definite diagnosis of the primary headache leaves much to be desired. In the case of daily headache lasting several years, both the primary headache syndrome as well as the superimposed drug-induced headache are misinterpreted.

- For pharmacological reasons, the administration of opioids and barbiturates in headache patients is not justified. This applies also to spasmolytics and mixed analgesics. Therefore especially fixed combinations are obsolete.
- The therapies appropriate for the prophylaxis of migraine, tension headache, or combination headache are usually started too late. The pre-existent drug abuse blocks any successful therapy or prophylaxis.

References

Ad hoc Committee on classification of headache (1962) Classification of headache. JAMA 179:717–718

Anderson PG (1975) Ergotamine headache. Headache 15:118–121

Diamond S, Scheubaum H (1983) Flunarizine, a calcium-channel-blocker, in the prophylactic treatment of migraine. Headache 23:39–42

Dichgans J, Diener HC, Gerber WD, Verspohl EJ, Kukiolka H, Kluck M (1984) Analgetica-induzierter Dauerkopfschmerz. Dtsch Med Wochenschr 109:369–372

Hokkanen E, Waltimo O, Kallaranta T (1978) Toxic effects of ergotamine used for migraine. Headache 18:95–98

Kudrow L (1979) Cluster headache. Diagnosis and management. Headache 19:142–149

Kudrow L (1982) Paradoxical effects of frequent analgesic use. In: Critchley M, Friedman AP, Gorini S, Sicuteri F (eds) Advances in Neurology, vol 33. Raven, New York, pp 335–342

Louis P, Spierings EHL (1982) Comparison of flunarizine (Sibelium) and pizotifen (Sandomigran). Cephalalgia 2:197–203

Lundberg PO, Osterman PO (1974) The benign and malignant form of orgasmic cephalalgia. Headache 14:164

Mathew NT (1981) Prophylaxis of migraine and mixed headache. A randomized controlled study. Headache 21:235–239

Mathew NT, Stubits E, Nigam MP (1982) Transformation of episodic migraine into daily headache: analysis of factors. Headache 22:66–68

Pfaffenrath V, Kellhammer U, Pöllmann W (1986) Combination headache: practical experience with a combination of a β-blocker and an antidepressive. Cephalalgia, 6[suppl 5]:25–32

Rapoport AM (1984) Kopfschmerzen durch Analgetica. In: Pfaffenrath V, Schrader A, Neu IS (eds) Primäre Kopfschmerzen. MMW, München, pp 47–52

Saper JR (1982) The mixed headache syndrome. A new perspective. Headache 22:184–186

Sjaastad O (1986) Cluster Headache. In: Rose FC, Handbook of clinical neurology, vol 4, Headache. Elsevier, Amsterdam 48:217–246

Sjaastad O, Dale I (1976) A new (?) clinical headache entity "chronic paroxysmal hemicrania." Acta Neurol Scand 54:140–159

Sjaastad O, Saunte C, Hovdahl H, Breivik H, Groenbaeck E (1983) Cervicogenic headache. An hypothesis. Cephalalgia 3:249–256

Tfelt-Hansen P (1985) Ergotamine headache. In: Pfaffenrath V, Lundberg PO, Sjaastad O (eds) Updating in headache. Springer, Berlin Heidelberg New York Tokyo, pp 169–172

Tfelt-Hansen P, Krabbe AA (1981) Ergotamine abuse. Do patients benefit from withdrawal? Cephalalgia 1:29–32

Weerasuriya K, Patel L, Turner P (1982) β-Adrenoceptor blockade and migraine. Cephalalgia 2:33–45

Welch KMA, Darney D, Simkins RT (1984) The role of estrogen in migraine: a review and hypothesis. Cephalalgia 4:227–236

Wilkinson M (1983) Treatment of the acute migraine attack – current status. Cephalalgia 3:61–67

Wörz R (1983) Effects and risks of psychotropic and analgesic combinations. Am J Med 75:139–140

Ziegler DK (1985) Tension-muscle contraction headaches. A review. In: Pfaffenrath V, Lundberg PO, Sjaastad O (eds) Updating in headache. Springer, Berlin Heidelberg New York Tokyo, pp 315–320

Psychological, Behavioral, and Social Aspects of Drug-Induced Headache

The Role of Behavioral and Social Factors in the Development of Drug-Induced Headache

W. D. GERBER, W. MILTNER, and U. NIEDERBERGER

Introduction

A number of investigators have reported that social and behavioral factors play an important role in the development and maintenance of pain-related behavior (Wooley et al. 1978; Fordyce 1974). A popular notion in behavioral literature on pain is that social reinforcement (i.e., consolation by relatives, friends, hospital staff, and physicians) increases the incidence of verbal reports of pain and overt behavioral signs of pain (Sternbach 1974; Fordyce 1977). Moreover, most investigators agree that receipt of analgesics helps to reinforce a patient's perception of pain. According to one particular theory, pain-relieving medication reinforces excess use of pain-related behavior by the process of immediate pain relief (operant conditioning) and moreover by the psychotropic action of most analgesics. The latter action results in elevated mood and mild euphoria. Termination of pain (headache) through the assumed action of the drug may increase the probability of drug intake in the future (negative reinforcement). Positive consequences result in a drug intake behavior (i.e., drug abuse) which is associated with increasing frequency and intensity of pain.

With respect to pain-relieving drugs, the hypothesis of reinforcement has long intrigued by psychologists, psychopharmacologists, and other health scientists. Surprisingly enough, strong experimental evidence for these assumptions is still lacking. Objective examinations of the behavioral factors affecting pain therapy would be very useful. Previous studies have examined only a limited number of the relative factors. Fordyce (1977) administered analgesics at fixed time schedules independently of pain complaints in order to prevent reinforcement of pain-related behavior. With this method he achieved improvement in the ability of patients to live with their pain by breaking the link between behavior and pain relief (a process called "extinction").

At present very little is known about the development of drug abuse in patients with chronic pain (Zlutnick and Taylor 1982). Research by Wooley et al. (1978) and Fordyce (1977) indicated that situative, cognitive and social factors, and especially the immediate social environment of the patient with chronic pain may play a major role in determining patterns of drug intake. This paper summarizes our own results concerning pain-related behavior in children and adults with chronic headache.

Departments of Medical Psychology, University of Kiel, Niemannsweg 147, 2300 Kiel, Federal Republic of Germany

Drug-Induced Headache
Ed. by H.-C. Diener and M. Wilkinson
© Springer-Verlag Berlin Heidelberg 1988

Drug Intake in Children:
The Initial Experience with Analgesics

An essential characteristic of migraine is the frequent familial occurrence. General behavior as well as pain behavior of children can sometimes be understood through the observation of behavioral patterns (modeling) of the parents and other close relatives. A common observation is that children may have easy access to drugs when one or both parents in a family take pain medication. The theory of social learning (Bandura 1969) postulates that children may be prone to imitate parental use of analgesics since these drugs may also result in an immediate positive feedback for the child (e.g., the parent immediately has more time for the child).

The question whether children acquire the habit of analgesic use from parents is investigated in a review of the history of drug-related headache, which includes retrospective as well as prospective analysis of drug intake behavior. Our initial data on the use of pain medication by children were gained from interviews of 223 adult migraine patients. A total of 95% of these patients had their first experience with analgesic drugs in early childhood or adolescence under the age of 15 years. To provide an empirical framework for continued research on psychological aspects of chronic headache in children, 22 young patients were investigated for specific headache parameters and drug intake behavior. Table 1 shows the essential characteristics of this sample. The children and their parents were systematically questioned concerning different aspects of their headache. For this purpose the children also compiled, with the help of their parents, detailed headache diaries over a period of 6 months during which they recorded different parameters of their headache as well as the medications used.

The results show that only 18% of the children took no analgesics at all (Table 2). The other 82% of the children, regardless of age group, took drugs regularly. During the 6-month period the 18 children used some sort of medication on 140 occasions (Table 3). No specific sex difference was apparent. Children with migraine used analgesics significantly more than children with tension headache (Table 3).

Table 1. Characteristics of child subjects

Patients (*n*)	22
Age (years)	
Mean	12.9
Range	9–16
Girls	10
Boys	12
History of headache (years)	
Mean	6.5
Range	2–11
Age at first drug	
Mean	9.2
Range	7–11

Table 2. Drug intake in children, based on headache diaries ($n = 22$)

	(*n*)	(%)
No intake	4	18
Intake	18	82
Analgesics	12	55
Ergot alkaloids	3	14
Others	3	13

Table 3. Frequency of drug intake in children during a 6-month observation based on headache diaries ($n=18$, f = frequency)

Classification of headache	Girls		Boys	
	f	(%)	f	(%)
Tension headache	24	19.5	25	16.7
Migraine	44	50.0	47	56.0
Total number of drug intakes	68	31.8	72	30.8

Table 4. Intake of analgesic drugs in children (frequency of tablets per month and chemical components; data based on headache diaries for 6 months) ($n=18$, f = frequency)

Brand name	Drugs per month		Chemical component	(%)
	f	(%)		
Aspirin*			Aminophenol derivative	45
or Boxazin*	35	36	Paracetamol (acetaminophen)	17
Vivimed	28.7	30	Phenacetin	28
Gelonida	14.8	15	Salicylic acid	39
Dihydergot*	8	8	Caffeine	17
Baralgin	3	3	Codeine	17
Ben-u-ron*	2.2	2	Ergot alkaloids	17
			Dihydroergotamine	11
			Ergotamine	6
Others	4.5	5	Others	59
Total	99.2	100	Total substances (n = 34)	

* Monosubstance.

Paracetamol and salicylic acid (aspirin) were the drugs most commonly used by the children (Table 4). The analysis of the diaries revealed a high correlation between the onset of headache and drug intake behavior in children. Pain relief (98%) and the apprehension of absence from school (88%) were the predominating motivation for the drug intake. The anticipation of school problems seems to be the main consequence of headache declared by the parents. Systematic analysis of parental behavior patterns indicated that anticipation of their child's possible school failure was the greatest problem.

Nevertheless, there was usually considerable parental uncertainty concerning their children's use of pain medications. On the one hand, medication was perceived as dangerous for their child's health and development and, on the other hand, it was seen as the only possibility to solve the child's chronic problems associated with headache (approach-avoidance-conflict). The danger of pain medication was especially evident to the parents since they were themselves frequent users. In summary, our results indicate that children suffering from headache begin frequent use of pain medication at an early age. Worries concerning school-related problems and immediate pain relief were the major factors influencing the onset of childhood use of analgesics. Our major conclusion is that effort should be expended to devise adequate methods for handling chronic headache in children (e.g., behavioral treatment, migraine prophylaxis).

Social and Behavioral Factors in Adult Patients Suffering from Drug-Induced Headache

Drug-induced headache is generally caused by regular intake of analgesics and migraine drugs (see Diener et al. this volume). How long a headache patient must take medication, and what factors determine the onset and course of drug-induced headache is still poorly understood and researched. A major question should be, why regular intake of higher drug doses occurs. Although some authors argue that pain relief is the essential reason for continued use of analgesics (Thompson and Pickens 1971), it is also certain that situative factors (e.g., work, marriage), social factors (e.g., expectations of a partner), and cognitive aspects (e.g., fear of career failure) play a remarkable role. An uncritical opinion of analgesics and ignorance of the dangers of their misuse can contribute to their abuse. By continued research we hope to be able to clarify these questions. It is for this reason that we have begun to employ the methodology of learning psychology (systematic behavioral analysis) and social psychology.

Drug Intake Behavior in Patients Suffering from Drug-Induced Headache

In an explorative study 27 patients suffering from drug-induced headache were questioned during their stay in the department of neurology. Table 5 shows the

Table 5. Characteristics of patients with drug-induced headaches

Patients (n)	27
Age (years)	
Mean	44.78
Range	24–65
Women	21
Men	6
History of drug-related headache (years)	
Mean	5.92
Range	1–26
History of migraine	
Mean	14.72
Range	3–40

main features of these patients. On average, drug-induced headaches were reported to have continued for about 6 years and 90% of the patients had used analgesics since childhood. The first pain medications were usually obtained on prescription (70%). Self-medication (22%) or receipt of drugs from parents (8%) occurred much less frequently. When asked about their use of analgesics, 58,3% reported that they sometimes took analgesics in the evening as a prophylactic to prevent a migraine attack the next morning; 40% obtained their medications from intermediaries (e.g., friends) rather from a physician; 25% had refillable prescriptions not requiring continued consultation with a physician. In addition to pain medications, a number of stimulants were taken. The most common stimulants were coffee (64%: more than five cups per day), nicotine (20%), alcohol (16%), and tea (32%). Barbiturates, sedatives, or hypnotic drugs were regularly used by 46%.

There were essentially two major reasons for the immediate or occasional prophylactic intake of analgesics and migraine drugs: pain relief (96%) and apprehension of losing onès job (54%). An additional reason was anxiety concerning family problems (29%). For 91% pain without pain relievers was unbearable, and 57% were certain that they could not perform their work adequately without an analgesic.

The responses of the patients confirmed the reinforcing nature of their medication. It was also evident that they were in a difficult psychological "double-bind situation." Although the regular use of analgesics lessened their anticipation of negative consequences (pain, job failure), 82% still reported severe complications, i.e., sleep disturbances (51.9%), circulatory disorders (53.8%), and of course long-lasting headache (89.1%). Correspondingly the patients had ambivalent feelings about drug withdrawal. A total of 81.8% were comfortable with their drug use only because of the support of their physician; yet 56% were sceptical about the success of drug withdrawal. A total of 94% initially expected quick and substantial help from their doctor and exerted considerable pressure on the attending physician.

In conclusion, the interviews based on behavioral analysis methods indicated a preponderant anticipation of negative consequence accompanying the use of analgesics. Nevertheless, it can be presumed that this anticipation is not only a major characteristic of patients suffering from drug-induced headache, but also a fundamental feature of headache patients. Further research was carried out to test this hypothesis.

Social and Behavioral Determinants
in Migraine Patients Versus Patients Suffering from Drug-Induced Headache

One of our assumptions is that drug intake behavior is influenced by specific attitudes toward drugs and/or by the normative beliefs of persons which may become confounded by headache problems. Relatives and friends as well as physicians can produce social reinforcement not only by attracting attention to pain-related behavior, but also by influencing the patients' attitudes toward analgesic drugs.

Methods

We divided 48 migraine patients into two groups: group 1 ($n=35$) included those patients using pain medications on less than 20 days per month (presumably not candidates for drug-induced headache); group 2 ($n=13$) consisted of patients using pain medications on more than 20 days per month (those more likely to develop or suffer from drug-induced headache). The characteristics of these patients are shown in Table 6. The difference in the two groups correlated significantly with higher age and longer duration of illness in group 2. No differences were found between the frequency of migraine attacks and the group characteristics.

At first contact every patient was questioned about his or her specific attitudes and behavior at the time when he or she began to use analgesics and migraine drugs. These questions were based on the "theory of prediction of behavior" by Fishbein (1967). According to this theory, the overt behavior of individuals or their behavior intentions (i.e., intake of analgesic drugs) is primarily determined by their attitudes toward the object and the behavior, their normative beliefs and the motivation to comply with the norms (see Table 7). Reference to this model requires information about patients' attitudes toward analgesic drugs, their supposed normative beliefs (parents, wife/husband, and physician), and their motivation to comply with these norms. Moreover, we asked about their concerns about

Table 6. Essential characteristics of the patients ($n=48$)

Variables	Non-daily headached group	Daily headache group	Significance
Patients (n)	35	13	
Age (years)			
Mean	39.9	48.9	$P<0.01$
SD	9.6	7.4	
Sex			
Male	5	3	NS
Female	30	10	
History of headache (years)			
Mean	18.6	24.5	$P<0.06$
SD	9.1	10.8	
Number of days with headache per month, mean	4.9	22.2	$P<0.01$
Migraine attacks per month, mean	5.1	6.5	NS

Table 7. Algebraic formulation of the Fishbein model

$$B \sim BI = \Sigma\, \mathrm{Aact}_{\omega_0} + \Sigma\, (NB)\, (Mc)_{\omega_1}$$

The overt behavior (B; drug intake) or the behavioral intention (BI) of a migraine patient is a function of (a) his attitudes toward performing the behavior (drug intake) (Aact) and (b) the norms governing that situation (NB) and his motivation to comply with those norms (Mc). ω_0 and ω_1 are empirical regression coefficients

Table 8. Measures of attitudes and normative beliefs with respect to the Fishbein model (examples)

1. Attitudes toward analgesic drugs: "analgesic drugs are:"

Good	+3	+2	+1	0	−1	−2	−3	Bad
Harmful	+3	+2	+1	0	−1	−2	−3	Beneficial
Wise	+3	+2	+1	0	−1	−2	−3	Foolish

2. Normative beliefs: "my parents think that I should take an analgesic immediately at the onset of the next migraine attack."

| Likely | +3 | +2 | +1 | 0 | −1 | −2 | −3 | Unlikely |

3. Consequences: "If I take analgesic drugs during the next attack the pain will be relieved."

| Likely | +3 | +2 | +1 | 0 | −1 | −2 | −3 | Unlikely |

the consequences of drug intake and about their evaluation of these consequences.

The actual drug intake (B) was registered by the patient in the headache diary. The patients were instructed to immediately enter in their diary specific headache symptoms as well as the quantity and type of any medication they used. Table 8 shows items in our questionaire. The data analysis was based on a regression analysis including multiple correlation coefficients.

Results

Of the patients, 85% responded that they would take a pain medication at the next migraine attack. The analysis of the diaries showed that they did so 77% of the time. From that standpoint the attitude of the patients toward drug intake appears to be somewhat ambivalent (see Table 9). The patients often had great regard for the perceived expectations of the spouse (55%) and physician (53%). The belief that the physician expects a given drug intake level is highly correlated to the behavior intention (BI) of the patients ($r = 0.52$; $P < 0.01$). Table 10 shows that the anticipated consequences and the evaluation of the drug intake appear to be

Table 9. Behavioral intention of drug intake and attitudes towards analgesic drugs and intake in migraine patients ($n = 48$)

Variables	+ (%)	? (%)	− (%)	$\bar{X}$	SD
1. Behavioral intention					
drug intake next migraine attack	85	3	12	5.8	1.3
2. Overt behavior (drug intake)	77	−	23	−	−
3. Attitudes toward drug intake in					
the next attack					
Intake is good	40	26	24	3.9	2.2
Intake is harmful	60	5	35	4.8	2.4
Intake is wise	17	64	19	3.8	1.5

+, Agreement; ?, undecided; −, disagreement.

Table 10. Consequences and evaluations of drug intake in migraine patients ($n=48$)

Variables	+ (%)	? (%)	− (%)	$\bar{X}$	SD
1. Consequences of next drug intake					
Pain relief	95	3	2	6.3	1.0
Side effects	90	3	7	5.9	1.6
Continuous negative effects	79	6	15	5.5	1.7
Capable of working	90	5	5	5.9	1.3
2. Evaluation of these consequences					
Pain relief	87	13	0	6.1	1.4
Side effects	6	13	81	2.2	1.3

+, Agreement; ?, undecided; −, disagreement.

the predominant factor influencing drug use. An analysis of variance for the various components of the Fishbein model showed that there was no significant difference between the two groups of patients. Moreover, there were no overall differences between the two groups with regard to attitudes or behavior.

Conclusions

1. Migraine patients showed a marked ambiguity in their attitudes toward analgesic drugs and drug intake:
   a) Positive attitudes toward drugs and drug intake result from favorable consequences (pain relief; capability to work; health)
   b) Negative attitudes result from unfavorable consequences (side effects; apprehension of continuous negative effects)
2. The intention of drug intake is determined mainly by these consequences and not by normative beliefs
3. No major differences in the characteristics of the two groups were found

Discussion

The present studies in children and adults show that analgesics already act as strong "reinforcers" during early childhood (see Table 11). Pain relief anticipated absence from school and job problems are the prominent motivating factors for taking pain medications. These results can be taken as evidence for the reinforcement hypothesis (Fordyce 1974). From the standpoint of learning theory, it can

Table 11. Operant conditioning in drug-induced headache

1. Positive reinforcement: the psychotrophic effects are reinforced
2. Negative reinforcement: reduction of pain by analgesics and migraine drugs is rewarded

be inferred that the temporal coupling between analgesic intake and headache can be strongly influenced by conditioning processes. This can also cover the induction of conditioned vasoconstriction as a result of the habitual use of pain medications (Christie and Kotses 1973).

From the point of view of learning theory, it is important to avoid or eliminate the temporal contingency in drug intake (see "pain cocktail", Fordyce 1974). The regular prophylactic use of pain medications without headache symptoms (e.g., prophylactic intake before going to sleep) should be avoided.

The results also show a strong ambiguity in the attitudes and beliefs regarding analgesic drugs. Pain relief and simultaneous anticipation of side effects lead to a psychological "double-bind situation."

From the point of view of social psychology, it is important to note that appeals arousing fears (side effects of the drugs, etc.) are not very successful. This phenomenon is also observed in other dependencies such as alcohol or smoking. Migraine patients, in particular, need strategies to cope with pain.

In order to avoid an increase of drug abuse and drug-related headache, it seems to be very important to elimate the contingency between reinforcement and use of these drugs. In preparation for withdrawal, through counseling is necessary to achieve a change in the patients' use of pain medications. The best way in patients with drug-induced headache is to immediately stop drug use and to switch to self-control methods such as sleeping or activation, acupressure, biofeedback, etc. (i.e., pain mastering). These procedures are, however, often ineffective in patients with severe migraine. Migraine prophylaxis (i.e., by beta-blockers) as well as different psychological strategies are very helpful since a contingent reinforcement of the pain relief process is not given with these methods.

The patient should be aware of the negative consequences of drug abuse (e.g., cognitive therapy). The involvement of the patients' social environment to support them during drug withdrawal is especially important. Prevention of abuse by awareness of the dangers and the psychological processes associated with regular drug use should be the responsibility of all the people involved and not just the patient.

Summary

It is widely assumed that behavioral and social factors play a marked role in the development and continuation of drug-induced headache. To examine this hypothesis, a series of investigations was performed with children and adults suffering from headache. The results show that analgesics and migraine drugs act as powerful negative reinforcers. Although pain relief and the feeling of well-being seem to be important for migraine patients, a strong ambiguity and sense of precariousness exist simultaneously in these patients. The physicians' opinions appear to play an important role in shaping the patient's response to drug therapy. On the other hand, information about the effective treatment of migraine attacks by these drugs is balanced by an awareness of the harmful side effects which contribute to the psychological "double-bind situation." From the point of view of learning theory, an important suggestion is to change the drug intake behavior of the patient.

References

Bandura A (1969, 1977) Social learning theory. Prentice-Hall, Englewood Cliffs
Christie DJ, Kotses H (1973) Bidirectional operant conditioning of the cephalic vasomotor response. J Psychosom Res 17:167–170
Fishbein M (ed) (1967) Readings in attitude theory and measurement. Wiley, New York
Fordyce WE (1974) Chronic pain as learned behavior. In: Bonica JJ (ed) Advances in neurology, vol 4, Pain. Raven, New York
Fordyce WE (1977) Behavioral methods of chronic pain and illness. Mosby, St. Louis
Sternbach RA (1974) Pain patients: traits and treatment. Academic, New York
Thompson T, Pickens R (eds) (1971) Stimulus property of drugs. Appleton-Century-Crofts, New York
Wooley SC, Blackwell B, Wingate C (1978) Aleting theory model of chronic illness behavior: theory, treatment and research. Psychosom Med 40:379–401
Zlutnick S, Taylor CB (1982) Chronic pain. In: Doleys MD, Meredith RL, Ciminero AR (eds) Behavioral medicine. Assessment and treatment strategies. Plenum, New York

Dependence on Analgesic Medication in Chronic Headache Sufferers: Psychological Analysis

P. Henry, J. F. Daubech, J. Lucas, and M. Gagnon

Being convinced of the harm caused by excessive and repetitive doses of symptomatic medication, if only in terms of the development of headaches, we have in recent years sought to develop a weaning technique by which we have monitored a large number of patients over long periods (Henry et al. 1985). Such prolonged follow-up before, during, and after weaning has enabled us to investigate beyond simple symptoms and more deeply than superficial monomorphism in trying to understand the determinant mechanisms underlying drug dependence.

Chronic headache sufferers (CHS) who depend on symptomatic medication seem at first sight to be the same. Their general profile is very stereotyped, whether they abuse analgesics, ergotamine tartrate, and/or tranquilizers. As in all CHS, there is clear female predominance, and the mean age is between 35 and 60. The patients' description of headache immediately points to tension headache, and only semiologic and evolving subtleties may reveal a subjacent migrainous pathology in certain cases. Occurring upon waking or at the slightest physical or intellectual effort, the headache is often a global one of the striction type, and of a pulsating nature at its height. It is usually a hindrance to daily life. It is only rarely an isolated phenomenon and is usually accompanied by asthenia, nausea, unsteady gait, insomnia, and difficulties with both memorization and concentration. The patient, who is sensitive to the slightest stress, is unable to tolerate the least frustration. Medication is reached for with the slightest symptoms, and sometimes even before and provides a rhythm to the subject's existence and that of those around him or her. What is striking is the fact that the body and the head are what the patient immediately talks about, and symptomatic speech often represents a screen to any relationship. Even if the subject admits to being tense and "nervous," his speech is "organic." "Just like the others, you are not going to tell me that it's just nervous!" is a frequent remark.

Overconsumption of drugs is often immediately apparent. The subject remarks "naively" that an intolerable level of consumption has now been reached. In fact, drug intoxication is only rarely mentioned spontaneously by the patient. Either hinted at the end of sentence, or minimized, it is put up with as a necessary evil. It is not rare for a spouse to underline the degree of drug abuse with a thoroughly disappointed or frustrated sigh. The "You can't go on like that!" repeated over and over again is often what prompts the subject to consult a doctor. Patients often indulge in hiding their behavior and in the clandestine use of analgesics, just like drug addicts.

It should be underlined that all the medication leading to drug addiction in headache sufferers (Optalidon, Propofan, Cephyl, Gynergen, Migwell, etc.) con-

Department of Neurology, Hôpital Pellegrin-Tripode, Place Amélie Raba-Léon, 33076 Bordeaux, France

Drug-Induced Headache
Ed. by H.-C. Diener and M. Wilkinson
© Springer-Verlag Berlin Heidelberg 1988

tain caffeine. Apart from tachycardia and polyuria, the "caffeinomania" syndrome characteristically associates impatience, irritability, nervousness, sleep disturbances, hyperactivity, and worry (Boulenger et al. 1984a, b).

A specific relationship seems to exist between caffeine and anxiety, more than with any other psychopathologic symptom. The search for the psychostimulating action of caffeine is for us one of the biological and psychological bases of the drug addiction process in chronic headache patient's, since it enables them to emerge from the drowsiness that excessive doses of analgesics and sedative psychotropic drugs plunge them into. The patients search for an intellectual and emotional erethism on a background of increased vigilance that caffeine procures could correspond to defence mechanisms of the maniac type; this will be discussed later.

Once evidence of overconsumption and a state of drug dependence is confirmed, a *proposition of weaning* will follow. Although patients admit to the need for weaning, they cannot envisage how this process could work for them. "If I don't take anything, it will be worse; My head will explode; I'll be sick all the time; I'll have to stay in bed for 3 days. I want to stop, but just give me something else." An offer of total weaning often causes an anxious exacerbation, and initial hostility towards the doctor: "I can see that you have never had this." In other words, the patient feels that the doctor cannot comprehend a pain of which the taking of drugs is objective and irrefutable proof. At this point, one must explain to the patient the intrinsic mechanisms of this pain: vascular instability, muscular contraction, inability of the organism to mobilize its own analgesic defences (enkephalins), events which are all caused by symptomatic treatment. The psychological elements are mentioned here and analyzed, but without any exclusive reference, especially during the first interview, since excessive psychology here would seem to the patient a denial of his suffering. During this physio-, and psychopathological explanation, the patient who felt abandoned starts to regain some confidence; indeed, a pain which may be explained is perhaps a pain which may be treated.

A proposition of weaning in a hospital environment and over a period of 12–15 days is then made to the patient and to his or her family. The weaning process is explained, and this leads to a contractual understanding between the patient and the doctor. A duration of 15 days has been chosen as optimal because such a period can be tolerated by the patient and is sufficiently long to offer tangible results. At this point, we do not request an immediate and definitive reply to the proposition, but we give the patient time to let us know what he or she thinks after quiet reflection. The patient's decision must be a positive and voluntary act which commits him or her personally. Detoxification can only come about when the individual has not only decided he or she wants it, but is also sufficiently mature to abide by the decision. A new therapeutic approach can only permeate under these conditions.

The specific time of weaning may constitute a chance for important psychic mobilization and also represent a decisive moment in the understanding of the psychological processes subjacent to headache, to drug craving, and to dependence. The period of hospitalization and weaning is also felt by the patient to be an intense moment in his or her life. The patient is playing his or her trump card and considers hospitalization and weaning to be the last chance. The beginning of this period is usually characterized by extreme ambivalence on the patient's part:

- The desperate hope that he or she will pull through, tinged with some scepticism
- Blind confidence in, but also aggressivity toward the doctor who forbids access to the miracle drug
- The fear of the pain that nothing will calm, but also the feeling of security that the hospital staff and environment offer

The schedule for cure is proposed in a rather stereotyped manner, since in our view a precise and relatively rigid framework seems to offer more psychological security to the patient than a nondirective attitude. During this period, the patient undergoes electrotherapy with Limoges current, the properties of which have been outlined by Daulouede et al. (1980) in obtaining weaning from hard drugs. The current is applied continuously over the first 72 h, then over shorter and shorter periods in the following 8–10 days. During this time, the patient and his or her family are informed that during the weaning period, the patient will not receive any symptomatic therapy for pain, however much it is requested; this unwritten contract is to us primordial. In some cases, if the reaction to weaning is exacerbated, particularly during the first days, the use of antiemetics and low-dose anxiolytics in the evening may be envisaged over a short time. In general, the absence of any drug therapy seems preferable in order to counteract the excessive oral craving of these patients.

Over this period, the patient is seen regularly for short supportive psychotherapy sessions. The goal of these sessions is to provide further explanations on the subjective symptoms experienced, to deal with underlying conflicts, to evaluate medical prescriptions, and to gather the opinions and impressions of the hospital staff. One or several sessions with the consulting psychiatrist take place here. This interview, which is announced to the patient in advance, is usually well accepted, although certain patients are sceptical about this type of intervention.

After the first few days, which are occasionally dominated by somatic and psychological reactions to weaning, the patients discover with astonishment, stupor, and sometimes delight that they have not taken any medication and that they no longer feel pain, or, if the pain remains, that it is tolerable. Their head is less heavy, less foggy, and the patients feel a new-found dynamism, a sense of freedom contrasting with the prison that was their previous dependence. Detached from the family milieu, and away from the conditions and conditioning of daily life, the patient discovers a new relationship with time, as well as a new self-image.

This period of hospitalization and post-cure follow-up often leads to better psychopathological understanding of the mechanisms involved in drug addiction and dependence. In certain cases, the trap seems quite ordinary and may be associated with psychological decompensation of a migrainous condition, since treatment of the patient's attacks has until now been given excessive attention in comparison to global treatment. Attacks give rise to other attacks, and the repetitive doses of symptomatic medication trigger new attacks. It is as if the patient were entering a new pathology without realizing it. Even in such apparently simple cases, the question remains as to why such a brutal decompensation takes place. Explanations, even simplistic ones, immediately come to mind: menopause, intercurrent pathologies, stress of life, etc., which are all apparently irrefutable elements, although none really addresses the question. These usual explanations are often just a priori assumptions which do not explain dependence, which is both a new pathology and a new way of life. The new dynamics, which finds its expression in and by dependence, is quite patent in the drug addict and is also present in the dependent headache sufferer.

An objection might be that drug addicts and headache sufferers differ, in that the former is in search of ecstatic pleasure while the latter is simply in pursuit of a nonpainful state. This forgets the fact that the drug addict's honeymoon lasts only a few weeks, and that his subsequent life is also the search for a nonpainful state. This would also be to forget the psychotropic, psychostimulating, and euphoric effects of many analgesic or antimigraine medications and their associated drugs.

To explain why dependence occurs, one could look at the moment dependence occurs and the way it sets in. The first particularity of initial dependence is that the patient is unaware of the antecedents leading to it. It is not a moment which immediately springs to the patient's mind when he is questioned. The replies on this point are only partial and only of the "vital events" sort. Most of the time, the patients themselves are totally ignorant of what has happened in those crucial moments. The following clinical case illustrates this sometimes surprising ignorance.

Mr. X, 30, came to see one of us toward the end of the weaning period. His headaches had become very intense over the 3 preceding years and had progressively reduced him to a state of relative social infirmity, which he himself called "almost depressive." For several months before weaning, he could only work, because once back home at 5.00 p.m. he would go to his bedroom where all was dark and silent and would renounce all social and family life simply because of the duration and intensity of his headaches. The medical history of his headaches was classic, with onset at 7 years of age, attacks spread over time and relatively tolerable, familial history of migraine, and progressive worsening over 3 years which could not be explained by anything in particular. The only thing he had noted was the progressive and ineffective increase in medication. He was most surprised to have dealings with a psychiatrist and proved both reticent and mocking regarding any suggestion of a psychological origin to his problems. After speaking at length about this reticence and when we, for our part, had almost decided that the interview would not be fruitful, he began to tell his personal history; without appearing surprised, he mentioned that his headaches had started at 7 years. It was at this time that his father had left his mother overnight, an event which was in no way explained to the child. The disappearance was abrupt and kept quite: "My mother just began to live differently," he said.

Then 3 years before consulting, he had had the idea of meeting up with this father, and against the wishes of his mother, brothers, and sisters, he asked the police to try to locate his father. He met his father twice, but they had nothing to say to each other, and he felt he had nothing in common with this man. Since that time, he had not seen him again. A short while after he began his excessive medication which was finally to bring him to hosital. This complex symptom-psychological movement interplay, apparently very clear chronologically, was related in very simple terms by the patient. However, throughout the discussion, the patient was not aware of the implications of the early events and left the psychiatrist as sceptical as he was at the beginning of the session.

This case report emphasizes the fact that addicitve behavior comes about through poor understanding of the underlying factors leading to its development and governing the imprisonment in drug dependence. Only a skilled practitioner is able to reconstruct the events surrounding drug addiction. The patient's scepticism is not surprising; it simply reflects the conscious mechanisms involved in the nonrecognition of the powerful factors underpinning his psyche. Through the history of our patients, it is clear to us that the development of dependence is often the patient's compromise to a situation of internal conflict that he lives through without necessarily recognizing it. Patients seem to misunderstand, at least in part, this conflicting dimension of their existence, or do not seem to realize it fully.

In this attempt to understand the psychological mechanisms underlying drug dependence, practitioners frequently observe a depressive or anxious component. However, in our opinion, the depressive component often represents the mental expression of the psychic conflict; it does not summarize it, nor is it necessarily an expression of its degree. The expression of depression or anxiety is simply the mental trace of the conflicting psychic situation. Headaches may be associated with the nonresolution of this conflict, while developing dependence constitutes the durable and pathological expression of this permanent state of conflict. Far from representing an equivalent to depression and anxiety, drug dependence is an alternative. It is only when dependence and self-medication can no longer mask the level of conflict that the patient feels the threat of depression becoming intolerable; this switchover to depression does not therefore underscore the depressive nature of the conflict but rather its psychological decompensation. It is often at this moment of decompensation that the subject chooses to consult a doctor. From then on, one must not fall into the trap of diagnosis anxiety or depression, leading to the all-too-easy prescription of psychotropic, anxiolytic and/or thymoanaleptic drugs, which themselves may cause a new state of dependence. It is only by seeking to understand the conflicting meaning of pain that its internal coherence may be perceived.

References

Boulenger JP, Marangos PJ, Patel J, Uhde TW, Post RM (1984a) Central adenosine receptors: possible involvement in the chronic effects of caffeine. Psychopharmacol Bull 20:431–435

Boulenger JP, Uhde TW, Wolff EA, Post RM (1984b) Increased sensitivity to caffeine in patients with panic disorders; preliminary evidence. Arch Gen Psychiatry 41:1067–1071

Daulouede JP, Daubech JF, Bourdalie-Badie C, Julian MJ, Tignol J (1980) Une nouvelle méthode de sevrage des toxicomanes par utilisation du courant de Limoges. Ann Med Psychol (Paris) 138:359–369

Guyotat J, Fedida P (1985) Evènement et psychopathologie. Congréss, Lyon, 18–19 November 1983. Simep, Villeurbanne

Henry P, Dartigues JF, Benetier MP, Lucas J, Duplan B, Jogeix M, Orgogozo JM (1985) Ergotamine and analgesic-induced headaches. Rose FC (ed) Migraine. Proc 5th int migraine symp. Karger, Basel, pp 197–205

Psychiatric Aspects of Drug Addiction of the Barbiturate-Alcohol Type

K.-L. Täschner and G. A. Wiesbeck

Headache in Drug Dependency

Headache and drug dependency are reciprocally related. Headache can, through the consumption of analgesics, lead to drug abuse and to barbiturate-alcohol-type addiction. In rare cases this mechanism can even result in morphine-type addiction. On the other hand, addiction, as is well known, can lead to chronic headache (Dichgans et al. 1984; Ladewig 1984). Here we want to discuss the psychiatric aspects of *barbiturate-alcohol-type dependency*. This is sensible given the fact that among drug addicts, the barbiturate-alcohol type is the most common.

Although drug addiction is one of the most frequent syndromes found in psychiatric clinics, it is also one of the least known (Ladewig 1979). The level of competence and awareness of the possible methods of treatment of drug addicts belongs for most clinicians to the more obscure specialized fields of expertise.

Phenomenology of Addiction

Addiction is a disease leading to the typical transformation of the entire personality. Addiction is synonymous with imprisonment. Drug addicts are at the mercy of a foreign substance, whose consumption can no longer be controlled by conscious and free choice. It is an advancing process which is dependent on a number of individual factors. It restricts the person's freedom decisively and continually, it is the cause of much physical, psychological, and social damage of the addict, and it requires qualified treatment. It can lead to permanent disabilities and to a shortening of the affected person's life span.

Addiction constitutes a form of pathological behaviour which penetrates and completely dominates every aspect of a person's life. Unlike, for example, bronchitis or gastritis, it is not an illness which strikes a given organ; neither can addiction be remedied through medication, rather it is a disability whose all-encompassing character resembles a mental illness. Addiction progressively modifies the very essence of a human being, including his or her basic convictions, attitudes, expectations and also his or her moral dispositions. In summary, all aspects that essentially determine one's behaviour are influenced. Addiction increasingly diminishes the range of a person's decisions, especially with regard to those related to the dependency itself.

Psychiatric Clinic, Bürgerhospital, Tunzhofer Str. 14–16, 7000 Stuttgart 1, Federal Republic of Germany

Drug-Induced Headache
Ed. by H.-C. Diener and M. Wilkinson
© Springer-Verlag Berlin Heidelberg 1988

In the course of its development, addiction takes over control of the person's entire behaviour. He or she is soon no longer capable of an objective and rational use of the medication.

Development of Addiction

These mechanisms can be demonstrated through the example of analgesic addiction. The initial phase can be a situation of emotional stress, often caused by some sort of conflict, characterized by headache, anxiety, uneasiness, and tension. The doctor prescribes an analgesic drug which helps at first. Its effectiveness, however, gradually diminishes with repeated intakes. Then comes the habituation phase, that is, tolerance. In other words, there is an increase in dosage due to diminishing effects. The third phase is that of addiction, when the patient takes larger amounts of the medication than initially prescribed. Most analgesics have the paradoxical effects of euphoria and a generally positive state of mind. The conflicts and problems, which initially triggered the use of the medication, fall into the background. The addiction takes on a course of its own. A common example of this mechanism is the development of addiction through the abuse of analgesics in cases of chronic headache, especially analgesics which contain barbiturates.

The last phase, is that of decompensation, characterized by inappetence, leading to emaciation, bodily decline, tremor, outbreaks of perspiration, ataxic gait, speech difficulties, and occasionally cerebral seizures. Social malfunctioning parallels this psychophysical deterioration. Social alienation and dereliction signal the final stages of this process.

Diagnosis of Addiction

We must always look for three components in cases of addiction (Wanke and Täschner 1985):

1. The underlying and basic disturbances of the individual; for example, headache, chronic pain, or situations of conflicts
2. The consequences of chronic drug use; for example, weakening of one's faculty of reason, long- and short-term memory impairments
3. Finally, we must determine one's susceptability to addiction (note: the extent of the addiction in relation to one's life is anchored in the personality structure and thus individually determined)

Apart from the psychological aspects is physical dependence which is revealed, for example, by the appearance of physical withdrawal symptoms when the particular substance is withheld. In comparison to the physical factors of drug addiction, the psychosocial components fade into the background. Addiction is less a psychological problem or a problem of willpower; it is far more a physical illness. The physical side of addiction is characterized by the term "tolerance acquisition." The body becomes accustomed to the given substance; it requires ever-increasing amounts in order to produce the initial effect. There are two explanatory models for this phenomenon:

1. The decline of the person's receptor sensitivity at the drug's side of action
2. Increasing acceleration of the metabolism of the foreign substance in the body (key word: enzyme induction)

The result is an increase in dosage. The total dosage per day soon exceeds the tolerable threshold of unaccustomed persons. This is particularly true for opiates, for which the therapeutic range is small.

Addiction Types

The World Health Organisation has defined seven different addiction types. For our purposes we are only interested in one of these, namely, the barbiturate-alcohol type.

The Barbiturate-Alcohol Type

Dependency of the barbiturate-alcohol type is characterized by an irresistable compulsion to continue taking the medication. In addition, there is a tendency for the addict to increase his dosage because of the considerable tolerance build-up, especially for sedative components. Along with the psychological addiction there also develops physical dependency, which leads to severe bodily withdrawal symptoms when the drug is withheld. This type of addiction can be observed in migraine patients taking barbiturate-containing ergotamine combinations.

Which Medications Bring About Such Addictions?

Next to alcohol (which is sometimes considered a medicament!) all barbiturate-containing substances are addictive, even bromine-containing soporifics, given the fact that prescriptions are highly abused. Also to be considered are barbiturate-containing compounds, which in part fall within the category of narcotics. Finally, methaqualone-containing soporifics, for example, Somnibel, should be mentioned in this context.

Other substances of interest are the benzodiazepine derivatives (Lemmer 1981; Radmayr 1982; Beckmann and Hass 1984; Böning and Schrappe 1984; Poser 1984) whose potential abuse, however, in light of our experience to date, appears small (Pöldinger 1976). This also applies to the benzodiazepine-containing tranquilizers, which are among the most widely used substances on the pharmaceutical market in the Federal Republic of Germany. Unfortunately, some headache and migraine combinations in the Federal Republic of Germany contain benzodiazepine derivatives. Their use leads to a general sedation and to an "anxiety-free tranquility in the sense that the user experiences a pleasant release from tension" (Schrappe 1976). In this context we must also mention Clomethiazol, which is likewise an addiction-producing substance (Keup 1977). Only in exceptional cases should it be prescribed on an outpatient basis. Yet such advice finds little reception within the profession. Cases of combined alcohol-clomethiazole dependencies are quite common and clearly result from irresponsible prescription practices.

What are most interesting for us here, however, are the nonopiated analgesics. When used routinely, they produce euphoria and generally improve one's state of mind (Wanke 1982). They contain, especially, the active ingredients propyphenazone and paracetamol, along with a lot of caffeine, barbiturates, and codeine. We can proceed on the assumption that roughly one-fifth of the adult population in the Federal Republic of Germany regularly takes such substances. Headache appears to be the primary cause.

Prevention of the Developments

It seems clear that we cannot, even in the light of the above data, avoid the use of common analgesics and migraine drugs. When prescribing medicine we should keep four things in mind:

1. We should limit our readiness to prescribe; for example, we should prescribe only to relieve pain
2. We should limit the dosage; for example, limit our prescriptions to the minimal dosage which is still effective and avoid gradual increases during the treatment
3. We should limit the duration for which the medicine is prescribed
4. We should instruct the patient to avoid the prophylactic intake of analgesics

Treatment of Drug Addiction

In conclusion we should remember that drug addiction is an illness which can be treated successfully. But such treatment requires special facilities which can accommodate the following four phases of treatment:

1. Initial contact
2. Detoxication
3. Rehabilitation
4. Post- or outpatient care and reintegration

Drug addiction cannot, as a rule, be treated on an outpatient basis. It is always a matter of long-term commitment. The central feature in this connection is "motivation." Only a motivated drug addict can be treated with any prospects of success. Therapy, against the will of the patient, is impossible. The prospects of successfully treating analgesic dependencies are not, however, as bad as often assumed; in any case, they are no worse than with alcohol dependencies. Through qualified treatment one- to two-thirds of the patients can achieve lasting independence from drugs. Such successful therapeutic results have also been confirmed by studies from abroad (Simpson et al. 1979; Sells and Simpson 1980). However, it would be ideal if we could prevent drug dependencies from the beginning.

References

Beckmann H, Haas S (1984) Therapie mit Benzodiazepinen: eine Bilanz. Nervenarzt 55:111–121

Böning J, Schrappe O (1984) Benzodiazepinabhängigkeit: Ätiologie und Pathogenese der Entzugssyndrome. Dtsch Ärztebl 81:211–218

Dichgans J, Diener HC, Gerber WD, Verspohl EJ, Kukiolka H, Kluck M (1984) Analgetika-induzierter Dauerkopfschmerz. Dtsch Med Wochenschr 109:369–373

Keup W (1977) Das Abhängigkeitspotential des Clomethiazol (Distraneurin). Dtsch Ärztebl 74:1903–1906

Ladewig D (1979) Abusus und Abhängigkeit von nichtnarkotischen Analgetika und Sedativa. Nervenarzt 50:212–218

Ladewig D (1984) Analgetikamißbrauch und Abhängigkeit. Münch Med Wochenschr 126:1201–1204

Lemmer B (1981) Benzodiazepine und Appetitzügler-Gebrauch und -Mißbrauch. Med Monatsschr Pharm 8:225–233

Pöldinger W (1976) Psychopharmaka. Neue Entwicklungen. Mod Arzneimittel-Therap 1:35–53

Poser W (1984) Tranquilizer-Mißbrauch und -Abhängigkeit. Münch Med Wochenschr 126:1205–1209

Radmayr E (1982) Die Abhängigkeitsproblematik bei 1,4-Benzodiazepinen. Therapiewoche 32:2838–2854

Schrappe O (1980) Toxikomanie. In: Peters UH (ed) Ergebnisse für die Medizin. Kindler, Zürich, pp 849–868 (Die Psychologie des 20. Jahrhunderts, vol X-2)

Sells SB, Simpson DD (1980) The case for drug abuse treatment effectiveness. Br J Addict 75:117–131

Simpson DD, Savage LG, Lloyd MR, Sells SB (1979) Follow up evaluation of drug abuse treatment in the DARP during 1969–1972. Arch Gen Psychiatry 36:772–780

Wanke K (1982) Psychologische und psychiatrische Probleme bei der Schmerzbehandlung. Therapiewoche 32:5550–5562

Wanke K, Täschner KL (1985) Rauschmittel. Drogen – Medikamente – Alkohol, 5th edn. Enke, Stuttgart

Pharmacological Aspects
of Drug-Induced Headache

Headache Drugs Provoking Chronic Headache: Historical Aspects and Common Misunderstandings

H. ISLER

Introduction

„Die größte Krankheit der Menschen ist aus der Bekämpfung ihrer Krankheiten entstanden, und die anscheinenden Heilmittel haben auf die Dauer Schlimmeres erzeugt, als das war, was mit ihnen beseitigt werden sollte."

"The greatest disease of men arose from the fight against their diseases, and the apparent remedies have, in the long run, created worse than that which was to be eliminated by them."

Friedrich Nietzsche was talking from experience; he had been suffering from frequent migraine since the age of 12, and treatment included silver nitrate solution, high doses of quinine, and aconitine. "Statistically: I had 118 days with severe attacks (in 1879); I haven't counted the less severe ones." In 1879, at the age of 35, he retired from his chair at the University of Basel because of his migraine. His descriptions are in no way different from those of our current patients (Holzhey and Isler 1984).

Patients

Primary headache is one of the most common practical problems. There is a hard core of chronic headache cases that resist usual treatment. Over 40% of these are associated with overuse of drugs (Isler 1982) intended for "instant relief" of headache; this drug abuse (Hornung and Gutscher 1984) appears to cause more chronic headache which is reduced by detoxication (Ala-Hurula et al. 1982; Isler 1982; Kudrow 1982; Saper 1983; Dichgans et al. 1984).

Usual Methods

Contemporary headache management is usually inconsequential: the functions of instant relief drugs and prophylactic drugs are seldom clearly distinguished. This strategic defect favors abuse, and relapse after detoxication. A classic example of such disorientation appeared as early as the seventeenth century: Sydenham (1667) warned against the use of quinine in malaria since suppression of paroxysms would make the disease worse, while, in chronic head and facial pain,

Department of Neurology, University of Zürich, Rämistr. 100, 8091 Zürich, Switzerland

Drug-Induced Headache
Ed. by H.-C. Diener and M. Wilkinson
© Springer-Verlag Berlin Heidelberg 1988

he recommended liberal use of opium, (Dewhurst 1963) founding a tradition in this vein (Sydenham's laudanum).

Drugs abused in headache are not mentioned in some standard texts on drug abuse (Blenn 1983; Wikler 1984), headache chronified from drug abuse is skillfully hidden in papers on drug-induced headache (Kohl 1983), and drug abuse is left out in about 99% of all papers on treatment of headache, migraine, and cluster headache, although it is probably the most crucial of all headache problems.

Auxiliary Method: Applied History of Medicine

The prevailing scarcity of reliable work in this field leaves us without landmarks since our otherwise successful "objective" methods fail to tell us where we are. New approaches are needed. Information usually discarded as obsolete may provide some guidance. Thus Mann (1984) proposed an inquiry into drug use from historical principles, and Isler (1986) recommended the application of history of medicine to these problems since we may be more confused by our machine-mindedness than our predecessors, who had nothing but their wits to rely on. For this project the historical background of current therapeutic attitudes was again reviewed.

Results

Evidence of abuse of pain killers is found in ancient literature dating back many centuries (Kuhlen 1983; de Chirino 1425). Warnings against worsening of headache by "too strong drugs" are found at least from the seventeenth century onwards (Maxwell 1679). In the nineteenth century blood letting, cupping, leeches, purges, and emetics were replaced by "modern" drugs in the treatment of headache. The list is suggestive of the best Borgia tradition, containing potassium cyanide (Trousseau and Bonnet 1832), arsenic (Buel 1808), sublimate of mercury (Martin 1827), aconitine (Burgess 1840), datura stramonium (Orfila 1819), secale cornutum (ergot) (Moretti 1862), digitalis (Muscroft 1872), opium (Adouard 1818), morphine (Day 1893), colchicine (Desparquets 1876), quinine alone or combined with tobacco (Richet 1832), digitalis, or opium, as well as sodium salicylate, potassium iodide and bromide, amylnitrite, carbon dioxide, and chloroform.

This violent pharmacopeia may be better understood when compared with the array of violent activities recommended in our own twentieth century, such as thorium treatment of migraine (Rothacker 1926), and nondrug methods such as radiation, intraspinal air insufflation, extraction of all teeth, hysterectomy, carotid cryosurgery, sympathectomy, intranasal and sphenoidal resections, occipital nerve exeresis, and oropharyngeal reconstruction surgery. The dominating principle of aggressive management is suggestive of the agitated behaviour of many headache patients who will bang their heads against walls, threaten suicide, or, in the same spirit, indulge in dangerous overdoses of ergot, barbiturates, codeine, and/or phenacetin compounds. A similar attitude appears to be celebrated by the popular term "painkiller."

After World War II, in Switzerland, abuse of over-the-counter analgesic compounds with phenacetin (Kielholz 1957; Moeschlin 1957; Horisberger et al. 1958; Gloor 1962; Dubach et al. 1967) led to chronic headache in over 30% of female workers in some factories (Kielholz 1957). Researchers focused their attention on renal disease; the chronic headache was explained as phenacetin hangover headache, or as a result of incipient kidney failure; it was agreed among nephrologists that the chronic headache *was a specific effect of phenacetin*. Ergotamine compounds were used to replace the phenacetin compounds: since there was a rational indication for them in migraine, they were believed to be harmless even if combined with barbiturates. Prescribed by doctors, and also available over the counter, they soon became a greater nuisance than the phenacetin compounds. On the other hand, those Swiss observations of chronic headache from analgesics with phenacetin had no impact on the international literature as they were usually not published in English.

Chronic headache, unresponsive to other drugs, and associated with frequent use of ergotamine was first reported in 1949 by Wolfson and Graham, then by Peters and Horton in 1951. In 1955 Friedman et al. wrote: "This danger seems to lie in an evocation of a medical paradox. Namely, in some patients the use of ergotamine relieves the headaches for which it is administered but at the same time leads to an increased frequency of these headaches." These early cases usually resulted from parenteral administration of ergotamine or dihydroergotamine alone whereas most later cases suffered from abuse of ergotamine compounds with various psychotropic substances (Olesen et al. 1979; Wilkinson 1983). Withdrawal of this kind of "ergotamine" decreased the frequency of the chronic headaches (Tfelt-Hansen and Krabbe 1981). However, after the pure ergotamine era, the additional substances in the ergot compounds were discussed by few (Tfelt-Hansen and Krabbe 1981), and ergotamine compounds were interpreted as "ergotamine" by most authors (Wilkinson 1983, 1985). Clinical or subclinical ergotism was thought to be the one and only specific effect that transformed intermittent responsive migraine into chronic intractable headache, perpetuated by rebound headache on withdrawal, and analogous observations on ergot-free analgesics were usually not considered in this context (Olesen et al. 1979; Wilkinson 1983), or disregarded after exclusion of other drug-specific mechanisms (Tfelt-Hansen and Krabbe 1981).

Ergotamine compounds were judged unnecessary in many cases of migraine and replaced by analgesics, very often in combination with metoclopramide and other psychotropic substances, in migraine clinics in Britain, Denmark, and Finland (Olesen et al. 1979; Ala-Hurula et al. 1982; Wilkinson 1985).

In 1982 Kudrow found that withdrawal of analgesics reduced the frequency of chronic tension, or scalp muscle contraction headache which

... generally occurs in migraineurs ... Thus with each successive stage of scalp muscle contraction headaches, increased analgesic use is associated with increased headache frequency ... These characteristics are analogous to those of narcotics abuse and withdrawal and strongly suggest shared mechanism.

He concluded that:

Frequent use of nonnarcotic analgesics may paradoxically sustain chronic pain and interfere with the therapeutic effects of tricyclic antidepressants by their suppression of central serotonergic pathways concerned with the regulation of dull pain.

He did not mention the other analogy, namely, to "ergotamine headache."

In 1982 Isler reported that withdrawal of combined analgesics, regardless whether with or without ergotamine, resulted in decreased frequency of chronic headaches. This was confirmed by Dichgans et al. in 1984, while Saper (1983) described overuse of both non-narcotic analgesics and "ergotamine" in the same paper, without commenting on, or discussing the obvious mutual analogy. The same noncommittal position had been taken in Germany in the 1960s when renal damage from non-narcotic analgesics was an important topic, for instance in Laubenthal's (1964) handbook on dependence and abuse.

Discussion

There is sufficient evidence of chronification of migraine and other primary headache by abuse of many widely different substances. The common denominator for the frequently aggressive methods cannot be found on a molecular or pharmacological level: they result from potentially destructive irrational behaviour directed against the obnoxious body of the headache sufferer. This attitude is not exceptional; it is very often encountered in disease and in the practice of medicine (Menninger 1938).

There is no reason to look for a single molecular property common to the many substances which, abused, will paradoxically chronify headache; if there is a common denominator, it must be the capacity of all these drugs to suppress the alarm signal, headache, quickly enough to enable the patient to avoid heeding it ("instant relief"); thus it is their very usefulness that prompts abuse.

Analogous phenomena are observed in the worsening of nasal congestion in privinism, of insomnia during abuse of sleeping pills, in the chronification of constipation by abuse of laxatives (Sleisenger and Fordtran 1978), and of idiopathic edema by diuretics (MacGregor et al. 1975). Chronification of quite heterogeneous intermittent autonomic dysfunctions by the very remedies applied against them appears to be common; intermittent dysfunctions are usually terminated by recovery of autonomic balance which is, however, blocked when continuous "instant relief" medication suppresses the feedback which is needed for the self-regulatory cycle.

This means that we are dealing with a behaviour problem in pharmacology. Behavioral pharmacology has been presented as a line of research (Seiden and Balster 1985), and it has already assembled evidence of drug effects modified by behavioral factors, e.g., rate dependency (Robbins 1981) where the changed rate of lever pressing by control animals appears to reverse the effect of a typical stimulant. Behavioral pharmacology has not been applied to the problem of headache chronification by headache drugs. Traditional "static" pharmacology has been applied instead, in vain. [1]

This is the method of the Eatanswill gazette, proposed by Dickens a century ago (Dickens 1836–7): in order to write about Chinese metaphysics, take the chapter on metaphysics and the one on China from your encyclopedia, and mix them up together. The Swiss physicians, narrowing down on "phenacetin," and replacing it with "ergotamine," and their American, British, and Scandinavian colleagues, focusing on ergotamine, and forgetting the analgesics parallel, showed how dangerous it was to jump to conclusions from preconceived ideas. The Swiss clearly succeeded in driving out their devil with a Beelzebub in the shape of ergotamine compounds with barbiturates, while their useful observations were practically lost since references in German cannot be read any more.

Conclusions

Frequent intake of *any* drug providing instant relief increases the frequency of primary headaches and blocks their response to prophylactic treatment. This condition which we may call *"chronic painkiller headache"* can only be treated by withdrawal of the pathogenic drugs, mostly by outpatient management, sometimes in a hospital ward, and, rarely, in a psychiatric ward. Usually withdrawal has to be substituted by prophylactic long-acting beta-blockers or calcium antagonists, and antidepressants. In order to change the pattern of dependence, behaviour therapy is needed; however, many patients are incapable of full independence; their passive dependence on drugs is often replaced by a residual dependence on the physician.

The current practice of narrowing down on artificially isolated details of this pattern consistently results in gross misunderstandings, and further iatrogenic damage to patients. Investigations are usually restricted to: References from the last 10 years and from English language publications; the properties of single drugs such as phenacetin, or barbiturates, or ergotamine; tension headache alone, or migraine alone; renal damage, ergotism, or psychosocial problems, respectively, as isolated problems; the psyche, or behaviour patterns, or the body's metabolism, as mutually exclusive fields of research. Such reductionist methods distort the natural history of the disorder. They are quite as pseudo-efficient as the pathogenic treatment of chronic pain by instant relief drugs. This ist not surprising since both are symptoms of the same urge for quick success.

---

[1] This reminds me of traditional psychological tests whose "static" methods for detection of brain damage and psychoses are applied in vain to headache problems which are functional and, hence, subject to distorting modification by treatment and observation. However, even in such conventional test batteries, headache syndromes arrive at a significantly different discriminance localization if compared to post-head-trauma syndrome, vertebrobasilar insufficiency, and heavy metal poisoning (Eskelinen et al. 1986). Furthermore, perception of various stimuli in chronic headache patients differs from that of controls without headache (Klein 1983; Appenzeller et al. 1984; Isler and Solomon 1984), and pain perception itself is modified by previous experience of pain (Eich et al. 1985).

Understanding of chronic headache associated with drug abuse has been lost more than once, and it has not been completely recovered: for most English-language authors, the problem of paradox effects of headache drugs does not seem to exist; they concentrate on those pure headache syndromes that are seldom encountered outside textbooks. Therefore any representative set of references must include German, French, Latin, and other non-English material containing old though not obsolete accounts of adverse modification of headache by headache treatment (Isler 1986).

In setting criteria for classification of headaches associated with substances or their withdrawal, further *inappropriate hardening of categories* should be avoided. Accordingly, there should be no heading "ergotamine cycle" or "codeine abuse" or "barbiturates" or "phenacetin" – as if there were specific chronifying effects belonging to any one of these substances. Applied history of medicine has shown that for too long we have not been able to see the wood for the trees. It should be sufficient to affix one label to the basic diagnosis, denoting "chronified by habitual intake of inappropriate substance."

References

Adouard E (1818) Céphalalgie périodique, combattue par le quinquina opiacé. J Gen Med Chir Pharm, Paris LXIV:318–325

Ala-Hurula V, Myllylä VV, Hokkanen E (1982) Ergotamine abuse: results of ergotamine discontinuation, with special reference to the plasma concentrations. Cephalalgia 2:189–195

Appenzeller O, Atkinson R, Kohner J (1984) Oral kinesthesia in scalp muscle contraction and vascular headache of the migrainous type. In: Rose F (ed) Progress in migraine research 2. Pitman, London, pp 257–264

Blenn K (1984) Handbook of abusable drugs. Gardner, New York, p 721 ff.

Buel W (1808) A case of inveterate headache, cured by arsenic. Med Reposit, New York, 2nd hexade, V, 1–3

Burgess T (1840) On nervous hedache from exhaustion, and its treatment with aconite. Edinb Med Sci J IV:95–105

Day W (1893) Severe occipital headache; subcutaneous injection of morphine; recovery. Lancet I:81

de Chirino A (1973) Menor daño de la medicina (15th C.). Edición critica y glosario. Universidad de Salamanca. Written about 1425, editio princeps 1506

Desparquets D (1876) Migraine de nature goutteuse traitée et guérie par le préparations de colchique d'automne. Rev Ther Med Chir, Paris, XXIII:231

Dewhurst K (1963) John Locke. The Wellcome Historical Medical Library, London e.g. p 94

Dichgans J, Diener H, Gerber W, Verspohl E, Kukiolka H, Kluck M (1984) Analgetika-induzierter Dauerkopfschmerz. Deutsche Med Wochenschr 109:369–373

Dickens C (1984) The Pickwick papers. Penguin, Harmondsworth, p 238. (First printed 1836–1837)

Dubach UC, Rosner B, Pfister E (1983) Epidemiologic study of abuse of analgesics containing phenacetin. Renal morbidity and mortality. New Engl J med 308:357–362

Eich E, Reeves J, Jaeger B, Graff-Radford S (1985) Memory for pain: relation betwen past and present pain intensity. Pain 23:375–379

Eskelinen L, Luisto M, Tenkanen L, Mattei O (1986) Neuropsychological methods in the differentiation of organic solvent intoxication from certain neurological conditions. J Clin Exp Neuropsychol 8:239–256

Friedman A, Brazil P, von Storch T (1955) Ergotamine tolerance in patients with migraine. JAMA 157:881–884

Gloor F (1962) Phenacetinabusus und Nierenschädigung. Schweiz Med Wochenschr 92:61–67

Holzhey H, Isler H (1984) Das Kopfweh der Philosophen. In: Barolin G (ed) Kopfschmerz 1984/ 1. Enke, Stuttgart, pp 103–113 (quotations translated by present author)

Horisberger B, Grandjean E, Lanz F (1958) Untersuchungen über Medikamentenmißbrauch in einem Großbetrieb der schweizerischen Uhrenindustrie. Schweiz Med Wochenschr 88:920– 926

Hornung R, Gutscher H (1984) Medikamentenabusus: Ergebnisse einer Repräsentativerhebung in der deutschen Schweiz. Drogalkohol (Lausanne) 8:3–24

Isler H (1982) Migraine treatment as a cause of chronic migraine. In: Rose FC (ed) Advances in migraine research and therapy. Raven, New York, pp 159–164

Isler H (1986) A hidden dimension in headache work: applied history of medicine. Headache 26:27–29

Isler H, Solomon S (1984) Impaired time perception in patients with chronic headache. Headache 24:160

Kielholz P (1957) Abusus und Sucht mit phenacetinhaltigen Kombinationspräparaten. Schweiz Med Wochenschr 87:1131–1134

Klein S (1983) Perception of stimulus intensity by migraine and non-migraine subjects. Headache 23:158–161

Kohl F (1983) Der Medikamenten-induzierte Kopfschmerz. Med Welt 34:25/1294–29/1297

Kudrow L (1982) Paradoxical effects of frequent analgesics use. In: Critchley M, Friedman A, Goroni S, Sicuteri F (eds) Advances in neurology, vol 33. Raven, New York, pp 335–341

Kuhlen F (1983) Zur Geschichte der Schmerz-, Schlaf- und Betäubungsmittel in Mittelalter und früher Neuzeit. Dtsch Apotheker Verlag, Stuttgart

Laubenthal F (1964) Sucht und Mißbrauch. Thieme, Stuttgart

MacGregor G, Tasker P, de Wardener H (1975) Diuretic-induced edema. Lancet, 1:489–492

Mann R (1984) Modern drug use. An enquiry on historical principles. MTP, Lancaster

Martin M (1827) Halbseitiges Kopfweh, geheilt durch Mercurius sublimat. corros. in kleinen Gaben. Ann Ges Heilkunde, Karlsruhe, 8, III, 2nd fasc:151

Maxwell W (1679) De medicina magnetica Libri III. Zubrodt, Francofurti, p 191

Menninger K (1938) Man against himself. Harcourt and Brace, New York

Moeschlin S (1957) Phenacetinsucht und -schäden. Innenkörperanämien und interstitielle Nephritis. Schweiz Med Wochenschr 87:123–128

Moretti E (1862) Storia di una cefalalgia scorbutica guarita mediante l'uso interno dell' estratto di segale cornuta. Gior Med Mil, Torino, X:392–394

Muscroft J (1872) Severe headache controlled by large doses of tinct. digitalis Cincin. Lancet and Obs XV:75

Olesen J, Aebelholt A, Verlis B (1979) The Copenhagen acute headache clinic: organisation, patient material and treatment results. Headache 19:223–227

Orfila M (1819) Effets remarquables d'une petite dose d'extrait de datura stramonium, dans une cephalalgie intense. N J Med Chir Pharm, Paris VI:374–379

Peters G, Horton B (1951) Headache: with special reference to the excessive use of ergotamine preparations and withdrawal effect. Mayo Clin Proc 26:153–161

Richet C (1832) Du quinquina en poudre uni au tabac et pris par le nez dans les céphalées intermittentes. Bull Gen Therap, Paris, 1832, II:427

Robbins T (1981) Behavioral determinants of drug action: rate-dependency revisited. In: Cooper S (ed) Theory in psychopharmacology, vol 1. Academic, London, pp 1–63

Rothacker A (1926) Weitere Erfahrungen in der Behandlung der Hemikranie mit Thorium-X. Fortschr Ther 2:692

Saper J (1983) Drug overuse among patients with headache. Neurologic Clinics 1, No 2:465– 477

Seiden L, Balster R (eds) (1985) Behavioral pharmacology. Vol 13 of Neurology and neurobiology. Liss, New York

Sleisenger M, Fordtran J (1978) Gastrointestinal disease, 2nd edn. Saunders, Philadelphia, p 1862 ff.

Sydenham T (1667) Methodus curandi febres. Gerbrand Schagen, Amsterdam (pocket reedition of the original of 1666)

Tfelt-Hansen P, Krabbe A (1981) Ergotamine abuse. Do patients benefit from withdrawal? Cephalalgia 1:29–32

Trousseau A, Bonnet G (1832) Recherches sur l'application extérieure du cyanure de potassium dans le traitement des céphalalgies et des douleurs nerveuses de la face. Bull Gen Ther, 2nd ed, Paris I:329–340

Wikler A (1984) Drug dependence. In: Baker A (ed) Clinical neurology, revised edn, vol 2. Harper and Row, Philadelphia. Chapter 21, p 1–73

Wilkinson M (1983) Treatment of the acute migraine attack – current status. Cephalalgia 3:61–67

Wilkinson M (1985) Ergotamine headaches. In: Carroll J, Pfaffenrath V, Sjaastad O (eds) Migraine and beta-blockade. Hässle, Mjölndal, pp 176–183

Wolfson W, Graham J (1949) Development of tolerance to ergot alkaloids in a patient with unusually severe migraine. N Engl J Med 241:296–298

Possible Pharmacological Mechanisms
of Chronic Abuse of Analgesics
and Other Antimigraine Drugs

R. Horowski[1] and A. Ziegler[2]

In the treatment of acute attacks of headache and especially migraine, drugs play
a prominent role. The antipyretic analgesics acetylsalicylic acid and paracetamol,
and, if these fail to bring relief, the ergot derivatives ergotamine and dihydroergotamine are by far the most important compounds. This conclusion is based on
published recommendations concerning pharmacotherapy of migraine and on an
analysis of the composition of preparations and combinations used in the therapy
of headache attacks. There is consensus that these compounds, when applied
properly, are effective in the treatment of an attack of headache or, when given
early enough, even in its prevention, although well-controlled studies which con-
form to the current rules of clinical pharmacology are not available.

The form of application is also of great importance, since absorption and bioavailability of these drugs are critical issues which are influenced by numerous
factors. This applies especially to migraine attacks because the motility of the upper gastrointestinal tract is slowed down (Carstairs 1958; Volans 1978; Ross-Lee
et al. 1983); therefore, the availability of an orally applied drug may be reduced
or retarded to such an extent that sufficient plasma levels are not achieved when
needed. This problem could be reduced, however, by appropriate pharmacological (metoclopramide, Volans 1975; Hakkarainen and Allonen 1982) or galenical
measures (effervescent drug formulations, Volans 1974; Ala-Hurula 1982) or by
using the sublingual or rectal modes of application in order to avoid absorption
in the upper intestine.

However, if drugs based on antipyretic analgesics or on ergotamine are used
regularly over a prolonged period of time, the development of chronic headache
constitutes a major clinical risk (Lippmann 1955; Rowsell et al. 1973; Andersson
1975; Tfelt-Hansen and Krabbe 1981; Kudrow 1982; Saper and van Meter 1980;
Ala-Hurula et al. 1982; Dichgans et al. 1984; Tfelt-Hansen 1985).

This untoward consequence of chronic intake of these drugs has been reported
several times but without real consequences for the theapeutic use. In the following, we will discuss possible mechanisms for the development of chronic headache
as a consequence of the abuse of antimigraine drugs. The discussion has to necessarily remain speculative since there is no relevant model of the phenomenon
of "chronic daily headache" in animals and since, for ethical reasons, no prospective studies in humans can be designed. A retrospective analysis, however, of the
duration and intensity of drug intake, of the drugs themselves, and of the conditions under which they were used depends very much on the subjective recording

[1] Clinical Research, Schering AG, Müllerstr. 170, 1000 Berlin 65,
Federal Republic of Germany
[2] Department of Pharmacology, University of Kiel, Hospitalstr. 4–6, 2300 Kiel,
Federal Republic of Germany

Drug-Induced Headache
Ed. by H.-C. Diener and M. Wilkinson
© Springer-Verlag Berlin Heidelberg 1988

by patients and doctors. We also have to consider that the population of patients with chronic use of analgesics and antimigraine drugs may be different from the general population; such a possible difference, however, cannot be established easily because these patients can be identified only after the chronic headache syndrome has developed.

Chronic headache does occur only after chronic intake of drugs used for treatment of acute attacks of headache. We therefore have to ask ourselves first why some patients start taking these drugs every day. The chronification of intake can be related to the antipyretic analgesics and to ergotamine themselves; however, since the compounds mentioned, as a rule, are taken in a combined form including other compounds as well, the combination or the additional compounds can also be the trigger of the chronic headache.

There are psychological and physical mechanisms which favor repeated drug intake and drug abuse. A fast relief from the painful symptoms can act as a positive reinforcing stimulus for repeating the therapeutic act which with time can become autonomous, i.e., drugs are used just as a routine even if there is no symptom, or due to fear of a hypothetical subsequent painful attack.

There is no doubt that the rapid onset of relief as a reinforcing stimulus plays a role in the development and persistence of long-lasting abuse, but we hesitate to consider this psychological mechanism as the exclusive etiological factor for abuse of so-called pain killers in headache. Chronic intake of acetylsalicylic acid and, even more so, of ergotamine at an effective dose is associated with relevant and unpleasant side effects in the great majority of patients, and we therefore have to consider additional factors which develop with chronic use and which reinforce chronic drug intake.

Among the physical factors we have to discuss first whether an enhanced pain sensitivity – and, thus, a high probability of a subsequent headache – is a necessary consequence of the acute suppression of a painful headache. Pain and stressful conditions are associated with the release of opioid peptides (for references see Hughes 1983). Hence, in the phase of pain relief caused by a drug, fewer endorphins and enkephalins are produced and, therefore, when the effects of an analgesic wear off, there is a relative endorphine deficiency associated with enhanced sensitivity toward pain. In systems other than pain perception, feedback mechanisms exist which can be altered by pharmacological means and which react to a transient pharmacological blockade with subsequent enhanced reactivity. Activation of sympathetic efferent fibers after stimulation of sensory afferent fibers is just one example (Bonica 1979), as well as, in the case of sympathetic activation, a hyersensitivity to catecholamines after all forms of long-lasting sympathectomy and a desensitisation after long-lasting sympathetic activation (Heinsimer and Lefkowitz 1982; Motulsky and Insel 1982).

In our discussion of the causes of chronic drug intake we cannot, however, restrict ourselves to antipyretic analgesics and ergot derivatives, because, in all the reports published, chronic abuse is not related to one individual substance, but to various mixtures of compounds which may have quite different pharmacological profiles. This is shown by the analysis of drugs taken in chronic daily analgesic abuse – whether this is manifested by chronic headache or nephropathy (Wörz 1980; Kudrow 1982; NIH consensus conference 1984; Dichgans et al.

1984). As a rule, combinations of antipyretic analgesics and/or ergot derivatives with psychotropic drugs such as caffeine and/or sedatives are used, the sedatives albeit frequently at very low dosage. So one has to ask what the relative importance of such combinations is in the development of chronic abuse in headache.

Several possibilities can be discussed:

1. All single constituents contribute to the wanted effect, i.e., rapid relief of pain. Thus, the combination would act as a stronger reinforcing stimulus. Such a therapeutic synergism, however, has not been proven for "classical" combination preparations, i.e., mixtures of antipyretic analgesics with caffeine or with sedatives. The widespread use of analgesic mixtures, their popularity or acceptance by the patients as well as their estimation by physicians is no proof of superior efficacy. A combination of several drugs gives a patient the impression of a sophisticated pharmacotherapy, tailor-made for his needs which he will thus prefer. Patients and doctors favor a combination of the freely available antipyretic analgesics with drugs which need a prescription because this, even if the dosage makes a pharmacological effect unlikely – makes the whole combination a prescription drug. This limitation in purchase alone will impress the patient as a guarantee of strong efficacy, and such an impression will most probably contribute to the psychological effects of the use of analgesics for the patient. Also, doctors might be tempted to expect a stronger pharmacological effect from prescription drugs – which also reinforces the ties between patient and doctor in a desirable way. Even if, with the present state of our pharmacological knowledge, a real synergism is quite unlikely, such combination drugs should be expected – as discussed above – to be a stronger incentive for repeated use.

2. The compound added to an antipyretic analgesic can have a dependence liability of its own. This is certainly the case with barbiturates added as sedatives; it also cannot be excluded for caffeine. A psychic dependence on caffeine is quite frequent; it is possible that some people prefer caffeine intake in the form of a tablet (e.g., while working) to the common ingestion of caffeine-containing beverages. For these purposes, people can take analgesic mixtures which are easily available. They are not really seeking the pharmacological effect of the antipyretic analgesic of such a combination, but have to take into account its side effects – be it chronic headache or nephropathy. As monotherapies are now favored in many countries – in part due to legal interventions – we will see in the future the relative contribution of combination products of antipyretic analgesics or ergot derivatives with psychotropic drugs to the analgesic abuse problem. At the moment, however, we must assume that the monotherapies, after chronic intake, will cause chronic headache.

3. Drug abuse caused by some euphoric properties of antipyretic analgesics or of ergotamine is highly unlikely. In experiments with rhesus monkeys neither acetylsalicylic acid (Hoffmeister and Wuttke 1973; Hoffmeister 1977) nor paracetamol (Hoffmeister et al. 1980) developed reinforcing effects. There is, however, a possibility that in migraine patients who are especially sensitive these drugs or their withdrawal can cause headaches, which is the reason why patients continue to use these drugs and form of a kind of vicious circle. It is known that overdose of acetylsalicylic acid (Vanecek 1984) can cause headache. An overdose of ergotamine, which is quite frequent (due to the low and quite variable bioavailability

of this drug), often not only causes headaches, but also nausea, emesis, and drowsiness (Horton and Peters 1963; Rowsell et al. 1973; Wilkinson 1984; Huzulakova and Dukes 1984), i.e., symptoms which occur during a migraine attack. Finally, headache is quite common after cessation of chronic ergotamine therapy, i.e., during ergotamine withdrawal (Saper and Jones 1986).

What has been discussed so far is that in the actual situation, no specific and generally accepted single mechanism can be found for the development of chronic headache. On the contrary, there are various mechanisms which can play a synergistic role in the development of drug abuse. We also have no reason to believe that the compounds combined with ergotamine and antipyretic analgesics – even if they contribute to the abuse – are of any importance for the induction of chronic headaches. We therefore consider these headaches to be a consequence of chronic intake of antipyretic analgesics or ergot derivatives and we therefore have to analyze which pharmacological properties of these compounds are likely candidates for the induction of chronic headache. Here, a problem arises, because for drug-induced chronic headaches we only have knowledge of the clinical symptomatology, but not of a possible pathological or biochemical substrate. In addition, we want to assume a common pathogenetic mechanism of drug-induced chronic headache, whether it is caused by antipyretic analgesics or by ergot derivatives, because clinical observation so far has failed to reveal any significant difference. This assumption, however, needs further clinical confirmation; it is supported by recent observations that in ergotamine-induced chronic headaches, antipyretic analgesics are helpful in relieving the withdrawal headaches.

Chronic Drug-Induced Headaches

Chronic drug-induced headaches differ from the headache in the course of a migraine attack. Patients describe chronic drug-induced headache as a dull and oppressing pain which interferes with a patient's performance more by its persistence than by its intensity. In this respect it differs from the typical headaches observed after a strong vasoconstriction with rapid onset (due to noradrenaline and stress), after vasodilatation (e.g., nitrates and antihypertensive drugs such as calcium antagonists or hydralazine), or after transient ischemic attacks, because patients describe these headaches as of sudden origin, pulsating, and severe. The absence of prodromes, unilaterality, and enhanced sensitivity to optic and acoustic stimuli differentiates chronic drug-induced headaches from the headache during a migraine attack. Both forms of headache can be observed together and are clearly distinguishable. Thus, in acute headache attacks, a rapid change in the vascular tone seems to play a crucial role, which justifies its description as "vascular headache"; in contrast, such a classification is not possible in the case of chronic drug-induced headaches.

As regards symptomatology, chronic drug-induced headache seems to be indistinguishable from headaches caused by brain edema, tumors, thromboembolic events in the cerebral vessels, anemia (including headaches due to high altitude), or forms of post-traumatic headache. Headaches as a symptom of brain edema or tumors have been explained as a consequence of increased intracranial pressure and subsequent activation of stretch receptors; such an explanation, however, seems dubious in the case of long-lasting headaches if one considers the physiological properties of these receptors. Since stretch receptors are differential receptors, they can clearly mediate headaches due to a rapid change but there is no basis to explain long-lasting continuous headaches.

If we look for an effect of acetylsalicylic acid which could explain its efficacy to relieve pain as well as its potential for inducing chronic daily headaches, an inhibition of the metabolic breakdown of arachidonic acid, i.e., an inhibition of the cyclo-oxygenases, is most likely. These enzymes promote the synthesis of cyclic endoperoxides from arachidonic acid if this acid is liberated from phospholipids by the action of phospholipases. The endoperoxides generated in this way can form, in part spontaneously, several prostaglandins, prostacyclin, and thromboxane. Many prostaglandins have a strong and long-lasting effect on the vascular tone, with some prostaglandins being vasoconstrictive (PGF_2) and others vasodilative (PGE_1). Their effects also depend on the different vascular beds, and therefore, inhibition of cyclo-oxygenases does not cause a uniform and general change in vascular tone (White and Hagen 1982).

Not only do we have to consider the disturbance in the physiological balance of the effects of several prostaglandins due to the inhibition of cyclo-oxygenase, but also the effects of leukotrienes which are formed at an increased rate during the inhibition of the cyclo-oxygenases (Hamberg 1976; Piper et al. 1979). The target organs of these so-called local hormones with eicosanoidal structures are mostly the smooth muscles of vessels, the endothelium, and platelets. Leukotrienes have potent actions in the microvasculature. In most microvessels leukotrienes act as vasoconstrictors, an effect usually more pronounced in venules than in arterioles.

A second target system is the endothelial cell. Its shape (and thus the permeability of capillaries) can be influenced, among others, by leukotrienes (Joris et al. 1987). Endothelial function and malfunction seem to be decisive for cerebral microcirculation (Rosenblum 1986). Leukotrienes are at least 1000 times as potent as histamine in causing plasma leakage, which is thought to be due to direct action on the endothelial lining in the postcapillary venules (Piper 1983). This effect of leukotrienes is probably prevented under physiological conditions by an increased formation of prostacyclin by endothelial cells which prevent these cells from changing shape (Dubose et al. 1987). During inhibition of cyclo-oxygenases, the protecting prostacyclin cannot be synthetized any longer.

A third possible mechanism could be a change in the balance of thromboxane and prostacyclin. Prostacyclin, which is mostly formed in the endothelial cells, prevents platelet adhesion to the endothelium, while platelet-derived thromboxane enhances platelet aggregation and adhesion to the capillary wall. Cyclo-oxygenase inhibitors will therefore alter this balance. A short-lived inhibition will have fewer consequences for platelet aggregation than a long-lasting one because the negative effect of cyclo-oxygenase inhibitors on the prostacyclin synthesis is short-lived while thromboxane synthesis by platelets is inhibited in an irreversible way. Thus, a short-lived increase in platelet aggregation (due to a reduction of prostacyclin) is followed by a long-lasting inhibition of aggregation (due to a reduction of thromboxane). If, however, inhibitors of cyclo-oxygenase, such as acetylsalicylic acid, are given over a long period of time, this difference is no longer of importance, and, therefore, enhanced platelet aggregation and disturbed microcirculation are possible. The consequences of a chronic inhibition of the metabolism of arachidonic acid are demonstrated in an impressive way by the changes occurring in nephropathy caused by prolonged analgesic abuse. Here, one first observes capillary changes followed by papillary necrosis (Bach and Bridges 1985).

Ergotamine – Dihydroergotamine

Both derivatives of lysergic acid have vasoconstrictive properties which are probably the basis of their therapeutic efficacy in vascular headache. Other derivatives of lysergic acid such as bromocriptine, dihydroergotoxine, and lisuride, which are devoid of vasoconstrictive properties, have no positive effect on acute migraine attacks, in fact, quite the reverse may happen in that these drugs may provoke migraine-like attacks immediately after the first administration (Cangi et al. 1985). This side effect disappears upon prolonged treatment, and even when used over longer periods of time, their use has not been associated so far with the induction of chronic daily headache.

Ergotamine and dihydroergotamine are vasoconstrictors but can reduce vasoconstriction caused by other compounds – a phenomenon which can be called "partial agonism/antagonism", but for which no clear explanation exists so far. As with the prostaglandins, the vascular effects of both drugs show regional variations and depend, as mentioned above, on the pre-existing vascular tone. In the case of dihydroergotamine, a specific and more potent effect on the venous vessels is claimed, which may be caused by a lower sympathetic innervation of the venous part than of the arteries and especially arterioles. The state-dependent effect of these ergot derivatives prevents us from describing a consistent effect on regional blood flow for all vascular beds and for all conditions.

These ergot derivatives also have an influence on platelet aggregation at concentrations of 0.1–1 μM in vitro. At therapeutic doses, plasma levels are in a range of nM concentrations, and therefore the effects on platelet aggregation observed in vitro may be meaningless if there is no drug-concentrating mechanism. On the contrary, after chronic ergot intoxications an increased number of aggregated platelets has been described.

The ergot derivatives ergotamine and dihydroergotamine are bound with high affinity to glycoproteins (Nimmerfall and Rosenthaler 1980), chemical structures which can be found in the gastrointestinal mucus but which are also a constituting element of the glycocalyx (Grant 1984) which adheres to the luminal part of endothelial and epithelial cells. The glycocalyx contains a great amount of sialic acid which conveys a negative charge to the surface of the endothelial cells; this negative charge makes an adhesion of corpuscular blood elements more difficult. The integrity of the outermost endothelial lining seems to be of particular importance for the function – especially the shape – of endothelial cells. As ergot derivatives have a high affinity to glycoproteins, they should be distributed preferentially in the glycocalyx. This assumption is favored by the observation in fluorescence microscopy that other derivatives of lysergic acid can be found preferentially in cell membranes (Horowski and Dorow 1981).

A strong, far-reaching, and high affinity binding of ergotamine and dihydroergotamine to apical membranes of epithelial and endothelial cells could explain why these compounds, when studied in isolated organs or in vivo, can have effects which do not correlate with the time these compounds are found in the medium (Müller-Schweinitzer 1984) or in the plasma (Tfelt-Hansen and Paalzow 1985). In such cases, the time course of the pharmacological response will not correlate with the pharmacokinetics of the drug as detected in plasma. They will be influenced by the dissociation of the drug from the membrane or, in case the drug interferes with the membrane function, by the time the membrane needs for recovery.

An accumulation of ergot derivatives at the level of vascular membranes could thus cause a disturbed glycocalyx function and a possible change in the responsiveness of the endothelial cells to other stimuli. Both effects combined can explain why ergotismus gangraenosus is associated with endothelial defects, a destroyed intima (Rall and Schleifer 1985), and the formation of microthrombi. Vasoconstriction and intimal lesions are involved in the impairment of circulation.

Hypothetical Mechanism of Chronic Daily Headaches

We cannot exclude changes in brain perfusion caused by chronic use of antipyretic analgesics and/or ergot derivatives such as ergotamine. In such cases both types of drugs would have effects on vascular muscles and the endothelial cells which would result in disturbed microcirculation. This would firstly affect cells with the highest activity and need of energy, such as the astrocytes which have a very high activity of Na^+/K^+ ATPase. Elimination of K^+ ions from the extracellular space is of great importance for normal brain function because neuronal activity releases K^+ ions from the neurons – an effect which, in view of the limited size of the extracellular space in brain, could cause a relevant increase in the extracellular K^+ ion concentration. If the function of the astrocytes, which exert a regulatory influence on the extracellular K^+ concentration, is impaired, then the transmembranous K^+ gradient is reduced and, as a consequence, also the membrane potential (for references in favor of this hypothesis see Bruyn 1984). Such partial depolarization could increase not only the excitability of neurons but also of structures which mediate the chronic daily headache.

Individual Disposition

There must clearly be individually predisposing factors for a patient to develop chronic daily headache when he is treated with antipyretic analgesics or ergot derivatives over a prolonged period of time. Chronic use of antirheumatic drugs which also inhibit cyclo-oxygenases has not been found to be associated with the induction of chronic daily headache. This also holds true for chronic use of dihydroergotamine when this drug is used in the long-term treatment of orthostatic dysfunction. However, there may be another explanation for such a difference: antirheumatic drugs may differ from analgesics used in headache in some other respect; for instance, it is also under discussion whether analgesics and antirheumatic drugs – in spite of being inhibitors of cyclo-oxygenase – can induce nephropathy to a similar degree. In the case of dihydroergotamine, on the other hand, problems of bioavailability could be a reason (Bobik et al. 1981) why this drug has not been found to cause chronic headache in patients suffering from orthostatic hypotension. These patients – in contrast to headache patients – will probably not increase the drug dose if there is no sufficient and immediate therapeutic effect.

In conclusion, we propose a hypothesis for the development of chronic daily headache which is based upon some assumptions (which can be tested in an appropriate clinical model):

– Chronic daily headaches caused by long-lasting abuse of ergotamine and analgesics do not differ
– Both groups of drugs cause chronic daily headache by the same mechanism
– This mechanism consists of a disturbed microcirculation as a consequence of a reduced brain perfusion

If a detailed clinical analysis confirms our first assumption, then it would be appropriate to test for symptoms and consequences of a reduced cerebral perfusion using modern methods. The concept of a similar pathogenesis would be supported by clinical results showing that patients have a higher risk of developing chronic daily headache if they use high quantities of both types of drugs, while their risk is lower if only ergotamine or an antipyretic analgesic is used. This difference could also be investigated by thorough clinical analysis.

References

Ala-Hurula V (1982) Bioavailability and antimigraine efficacy of effervescent ergotamine. Headache 22:167–170
Ala-Hurula V, Myllylä V, Hokkanen E (1982) Ergotamine abuse: results of ergotamine discontinuance with special reference to plasma concentrations. Cephalalgia 2:189–195
Andersson PG (1975) Ergotamine headache. Headache 15:118–121
Bach PH, Bridges JW (1985) Chemically induced renal papillary necrosis and upper urothelial carcinoma. CRC Crit Rev Toxicol 15:217–329
Bobik A, Jennings G, Skews H, Esler M, McLean A (1981) Low oral bioavailability of dihydroergotamine and first pass extraction on patients with orthostatic hypotension. Clin Pharmacol Ther 30:673–679
Bonica JJ (1979) In: Bonica JJ, Liebeskind DG, Abbe-Fessard DG (eds) Advances in pain research and therapy, vol 3. Raven, New York, p 141
Bruyn GW (1984) The pathomechanism of migraine as a basis for pharmacotherapy: a clinician's epilogue. In: Amery WK, van Nueten JM, Wauquier A (eds) The pharmacological basis of migraine therapy. Pitman, London, pp 267–278

Cangi F, Fanciullacci M, Pietrini U, Boccuni M, Sicuteri F (1985) Emergence of pain and extra-pain phenomena from dopaminomimetics in migraine. In: Pfaffenrath V, Lundberg P-O, Sjaastad O (eds) Updating in headache. Springer, Berlin Heidelberg New York, pp 276–280

Carstairs LS (1958) Headache and gastric emptying time. Proc R Soc Med 51:790–793

Dichgans J, Diener HC, Gerber WD, Verspohl EJ, Kukiolka H, Kluck M (1984) Analgetika-induzierter Dauerkopfschmerz. Dtsch Med Wochenschr 109:369–373

Dubose DA, Shepro D, Hechtman HB (1987) Correlation among endothelial cell shape, F-actin arrangement, and prostacyclin synthesis. Life Sci 40:447–453

Grant CWM (1984) Cell surface structural implications of some experiments with isolated gly-colipids and glycoproteins. Can J Biochem Cell Biol 62:1151–1157

Hakkarainen H, Allonen H (1982) Ergotamine vs metoclopramide vs their combination in acute migraine attacks. Headache 22:10–12

Hamberg M (1976) On the formation of thromboxane B_2 and 12-L-hydroxy-5,8,10,14-eicosate-traenoic acid (12 ho-20:4) in tissues from the guinea pig. Biochem Biophys Acta 431:651–654

Heinsimer JA, Lefkowitz RJ (1982) Adrenergic receptors: biochemistry, regulation, molecular mechanisms and clinical implications. J Lab Clin Med 100:641–658

Hoffmeister F (1977) Self-administration of codeine plus acetylsalicylic acid in rhesus monkeys with unlimited access to the drugs. Pharmacol Biochem Behav 6:179–182

Hoffmeister F, Wuttke W (1973) Self-administration of acetylsalicylic acid and combinations with codeine and caffeine in rhesus monkeys. J Pharmacol Exp Ther 186:266–275

Hoffmeister F, Dycka J, Rämsch K (1980) Intragastric self-administration in the rhesus monkey: a comparison of the reinforcing effects of codeine, phenacetin and paracetamol. J Pharmacol Exp Ther 214:213–218

Hokkanen E, Waltimo O, Kallanranta T (1978) Toxic effects of ergotamine used for migraine. Headache 18:95

Horowski R, Dorow R (1981) Influence of estradiol and other gonadal steroids on central effects of lisuride and comparable ergot derivatives. In: Wuttke W, Horowski R (eds) Gonadal ste-roids and brain function. Springer, Berlin Heidelberg New York, pp 169–181

Horton BT, Peters GA (1963) Clinical manifestations of excessive use of ergotamine prepara-tions and manifestations of withdrawal effect. Report of 52 cases. Headache 2:214–227

Hughes J (1983) Biogenesis, release and inactivation of enkephalins and dynorphins. Br Med Bull 39:17–24

Huzulakova I, Dukes MNG (1984) Drugs affecting autonomic functions of the extrapyramidal system. In: Dukes MNG (ed) Meyler's side effects of drugs. Elsevier, Amsterdam, p 244

Joris I, Majno G, Corey EJ, Lewis RA (1987) The mechanism of vascular leakage induced by leukotriene E_4. Endothelial contraction. Am J Pathol 126:19–24

Kudrow L (1982) Paradoxical effects of frequent analgesic use. Adv Neurol 33:335–341

Lippman CW (1955) Characteristic headache resulting from prolonged use of ergot derivatives. J Nerv Ment Dis 121:270–273

Motulsky HJ, Insel PA (1982) Adrenergic receptors in man. Direct identification, physiological regulation, and clinical alterations. N Engl J Med 307:18–29

Müller-Schweinitzer E (1984) What is known about the action of dihydroergotamine on the vasculature in man. Int J Clin Pharmacol Ther Toxicol 22:677–682

NIH consensus conference (1984) Analgesic associated kidney disease. JAMA 251:3123–3125

Nimmerfall F, Rosenthaler J (1980) Significance of the goblet-cell mucin layer, the outermost luminal barrier to passage through the gut wall. Biochem Biophys Res Commun 94:960–966

Piper PJ (1983) Pharmacology of leukotrienes. Br Med Bull 39:255–259

Piper PJ, Tippins JR, Morris HR, Taylor GW (1979) Arachidonic acid metabolism and SRS-A. In: Brune K, Baggiolini M (eds) Inflammation and thrombosis. Birkhaeuser, Basel, pp 37–48

Rall TW, Schleifer LS (1985) Drugs affecting uterine motility. In: Gilmann AG, Goodman LS, Rall TW, Murad F (eds) The pharmacological basis of therapeutics. Macmillan, New York, p 938

Rose FC, Wilkinson M (1976) Ergotamine tartrate overdose. Br Med J I:525

Rosenblum WI (1986) Biology of disease. Aspects of endothelial malfunction and function in cerebral microvessels. Lab Invest 55:252–268

Ross-Lee LM, Eadie MJ, Hazlewood V, Bochner F, Tyrer JH (1983) Aspirin pharmacokinetics, the effect of metoclopramide. Eur J Clin Pharmacol 83:777–785

Rowsell AR, Neylan C, Wilkinson M (1973) Ergotamine induced headache in migraine patients. Headache 13:65–67

Saper JR, Jones JM (1986) Ergotamine tartrate dependency: features and possible mechanisms. Clin Neuropharmacol 9:244–256

Saper JR, van Meter MJ (1980) Ergotamine habituation: analysis and profile. Headache 20:159

Tfelt-Hansen P (1985) Ergotamine headache. In: Pfaffenrath V, Lundberg P-O, Sjaastad O (eds) Updating in headache. Springer, Berlin Heidelberg New York, pp 169–172

Tfelt-Hansen P, Krabbe AA (1981) Ergotamine abuse. Do patients benefit from withdrawal? Cephalagia 1:29–32

Tfelt-Hansen P, Paalzow L (1985) Intramuscular ergotamine: plasma levels and dynamic activity. Clin Pharmacol Ther 37:29–35

Vanecek J (1984) Antipyretic analgesics. In: Dukes MNG (ed) Meyler's side effects of drugs. Elsevier, Amsterdam, p 137

Volans GN (1974) The absorption of effervescent aspirin during migraine. Br Med J 1974:265–269

Volans GN (1975) The effect of metoclopramide on the absorption of effervescent aspirin in migraine. Br J Clin Pharmacol 2:57–63

Volans GN (1978) Migraine and drug absorption. Clin Pharmacokinet 3:313–318

White RP, Hagen AA (1982) Cerebrovascular actions of prostaglandins. Pharmacol Ther 18:313–331

Wilkinson M (1984) Adverse reactions to drugs used in the treatment of migraine. Adv Drug Reaction Bull 108:400–403

Wörz R (1980) Abuse and paradoxical effects of analgesic drug mixtures. Br J Clin Pharmacol 10:391–393

Clinical Pharmacology of Ergotamine. An Overview

P. Tfelt-Hansen

Introduction

Ergotamine is still the drug of choice in the treatment of severe migraine attacks where it is effective in 80% of patients (Rall and Schleifer 1980). Its use is, however, often hampered by side effects (nausea and/or vomiting, leg cramps, paresthesias in the extremities, and abdominal pain) which occur in 10%–20% of patients after a *single* therapeutic dose (Rall and Schleifer 1980). Furthermore, *chronic* daily intake of ergotamine can cause ergotamine headache and dependence (Rowsell et al. 1973; Andersson 1975). In order to avoid or minimize these side effects, a thorough knowledge of the clinical pharmacology of ergotamine is needed.

Clinical pharmacology of a drug includes both pharmacokinetics – "what the body does to the drug" – and pharmacodynamics – "what the drug does to the body" – and in recent years both these aspects of the clinical pharmacology of ergotamine have been investigated. This paper will give an overview of these results. Finally, some clinical implications will be discussed.

Pharmacokinetics of Ergotamine

The high specific activity of ergotamine and its chemical unstability have until recently hampered the development of methods for measuring the drug in plasma, where the concentration of ergotamine is below 1 ng/ml after normal therapeutic doses. The pharmacokinetics – absorption, distribution, and rate of metabolism – of ergotamine has so far been studied with tritium-labeled ergotamine (Aellig and Nüesch 1977), with a radioimmunoassay (Ala-Hurula et al. 1979 a, b), with a high-performance liquid chromatografic (HPLC) method (Ekbom et al. 1983; Ibraheem et al. 1982, 1983, 1985), and quite recently with a mass spectrometry method (Haering et al. 1985).

In the first study, tritium-labeled ergotamine was administered i.v. and orally to healthy volunteers (Aellig and Nüesch 1977). The radioactivity in plasma declined in two phases with half-lives of 2 and 21 h, respectively. The lack of distinction between parent drug and metabolites makes interpretation of the results difficult. The study did, however, produce one substantial result: it could be demonstrated that 66% of ergotamine administered orally is absorbed. That a drug is

---

Department of Neurology, Københavns amts sygehus i Gentofte, 2900 Hellerup, Denmark

Drug-Induced Headache
Ed. by H.-C. Diener and M. Wilkinson
© Springer-Verlag Berlin Heidelberg 1988

absorbed is, however, not equal to a good bioavailability, as will be discussed later.

Ergotamine in plasma was measured with a radioimmunoassay after single i.m., oral, and rectal doses in volunteers (Ala-Hurula et al. 1979a) and after repeated oral and rectal doses in migraine patients (Ala-Hurula et al. 1979b). The main results of these studies were the very low concentration of ergotamine in plasma after oral and rectal doses compared to i.m. administration, indicating a low oral and rectal bioavailability of ergotamine. One peculiar result in both studies was the appearance of a second peak of measurable ergotamine after 48 h and later, indicating the risk of accumulation of ergotamine or metabolites. In contrast, in a later study using the same radioimmunoassay we could not find such a second peak when plasma concentrations were followed for 5 days after a single i.m. injection (Tfelt-Hansen, unpublished work). The reason for the second peak observed in the first studies with the radioimmunoassay (Ala-Hurula et al. 1979a, b) remains obscure. If it is due to some metabolites redistributing in the body, they do not seem to have any pharmacodynamic effect since the vasoconstrictory effect of a single dose of ergotamine has disappeared after 48 h (Tfelt-Hansen et al. 1980).

The HPLC method with fluorescence detection for determination of ergotamine in plasma has a detection limit of 100 pg/ml (Edlund 1981). The main advantage of the method is its specificity. A solution of ergotamine contains two stereo-chemical isomers: 60% ergotamine and 40% ergotaminine, and ergotaminine is without pharmacological effects (Schlientz et al. 1961). The HPLC easily separates these two isomers (Edlund 1981), wherease the radioimmunoassay cannot distinguish between the two isomers (Rosenthaler et al. 1984). Using the HPLC method for determining ergotamine, we have investigated the basic kinetic parameters: volume of distribution and clearance of ergotamine after i.v. injection of the drug (Ekbom et al. 1983; Ibraheem et al. 1982, 1985). Ergotamine is quickly distributed with a half-life of 2–3 min and an elimination half-life of 2 h. Ergotamine is cleared extensively during the passage through the liver – an extraction ratio greater than 0.75 was found (Tfelt-Hansen 1986). The blood clearance is 2.1 l per minute, that is, greater than the hepatic blood flow, indicating that ergotamine must also be metabolized outside the liver (Ibraheem et al. 1985). Furthermore, plasma concentrations were measured after administration of ergotamine as i.m. injections, regular tablets, effervescent tablets, suppositories, rectal solution, and after administration with an inhalation device (Ekbom et al. 1983; Ibraheem et al. 1982, 1983). The i.m. bioavailability was 47%, but for all other routes of administration the ergotamine concentrations were so near the detection limit for the method that only estimates of bioavailability could be given (see Table 1). Rectal solution of ergotamine and inhalation of the drug did, however, produce measurable peak levels immediately after administration (Figs. 1 and 2).

The newly introduced mass spectrometric method for determination of ergotamine in plasma has a detection limit of 10 pg/ml (Haering et al. 1985), but can probably not distinguish between ergotamine and ergotaminine. This very sensitive method has so far been used in the comparison of oral and rectal administration of ergotamine where the HPLC method has not been sensitive enough

Table 1. Summary of pharmacokinetics of ergotamine by different routes of administration. (Data from Ibraheem et al. 1982, 1983, 1985; Ekbom et al. 1983)

Route	Dose (mg)	Appears quickly in blood	Bioavailability[a] (%)
Intravenous	0.25–0.5	+	100
Intramuscular	0.5	+	47
Tablets	2	−	< 1
Effervescent tablets	2	−	< 1
Sublingual tablets	2	−	< 1
Suppositories	2	−	1–2
Rectal solution	2	+	1–3
Inhalation device	2.16	+	1–3

[a] Due to the extremely low concentrations of ergotamine by routes other than injection, formal estimations of bioavailability cannot be performed and the values given should only be considered as qualified guesses.

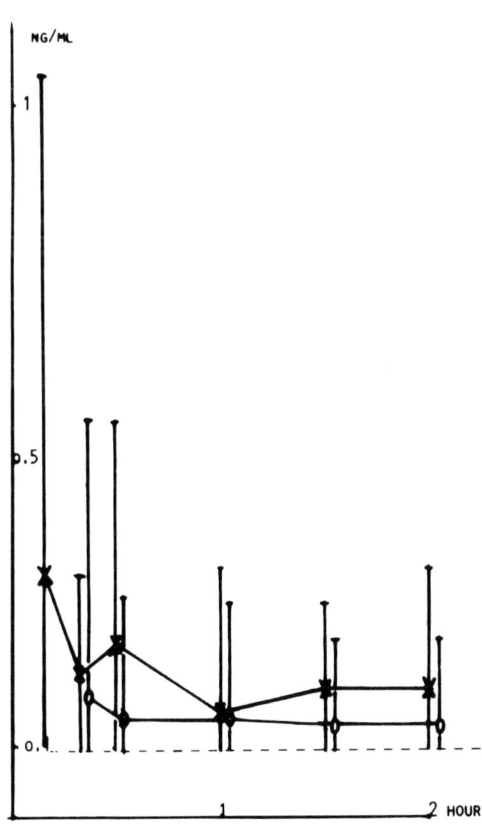

Fig. 1. Plasma levels of ergotamine after 2 mg ergotamine tartrate given as a suppository (*o*) and as a rectal solution (*x*) in seven migraine patients. Means and ranges are given. Note the very low concentrations, and that only the rectal solution resulted in a quick absorption of ergotamine. (Data from Ibraheem et al. 1983)

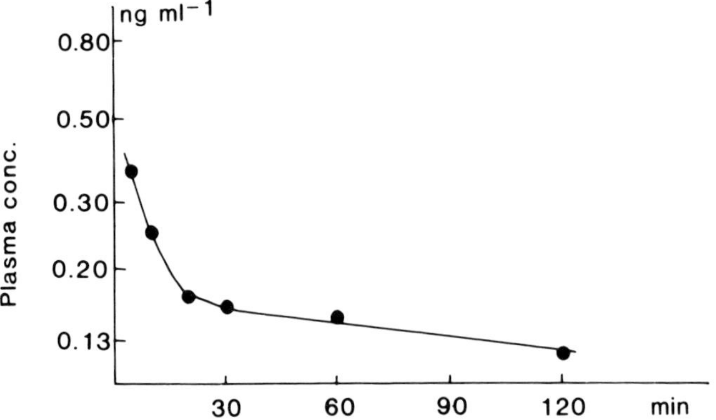

Fig. 2. Mean plasma concentrations of ergotamine after inhalation of 2.16 mg ergotamine tartrate in eight cluster headache patients. Note the instantaneous absorption of a small fraction of the administered ergotamine. (From Ekbom K et al. 1983)

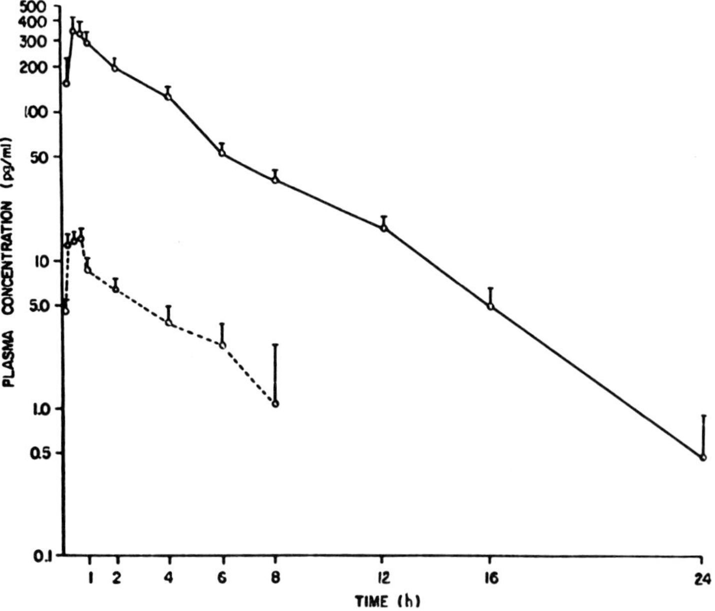

Fig. 3. Mean plasma concentrations measured following single 2 mg oral (– – –) and rectal (———) doses of ergotamine in healthy volunteers (mean ± SEM). (From Sanders et al. 1986)

(Sanders et al. 1986). The results shown in Fig. 3 demonstrate that ergotamine has a 20-fold higher area under the curve after rectal than after oral administration. The extremely low concentration of ergotamine after oral administration despite a reasonable absorption of 66% (Aellig and Nüesch 1977) must be due to an extensive first passage effect in the liver. That the bioavailability is 20 times higher after rectal than after oral administration must be due to some ergotamine being absorbed directly into the systemic circulation, thereby escaping the first passage effect in the liver.

Table 1 gives a summary of the pharmacokinetics of ergotamine. Except for i.m. injection, the bioavailability is only a few percent and for oral administration below 1%. Oral ergotamine in a dose of 1 mg has, however, been found effective in the treatment of migraine attacks (Hakkarainen et al. 1979). Could this be due to active metabolites? The problem of active metabolites of the ergot alkaloids has gained renewed interest since it was recently shown that both dihydroergotamine (Maurer and Frick 1984; Aellig 1984) and methysergide (Bredberg et al. 1986; Tfelt-Hansen et al. 1987) have active metabolites in man. My personal opinion is that active metabolites are probably involved in the therapeutic effect of ergotamine which is administered orally and to some extent rectally. Until the metabolites have been isolated and tested for pharmacological effects, the question must, however, remain open.

Pharmacodynamics of Ergotamine

The principal action of ergotamine is vasoconstriction, and since the work of Graham and Wolff (1938), this vasoconstrictory effect has been regarded as the pharmacological effect responsible for the therapeutic efficacy of ergotamine. Recently, however, it has been suggested that the efficacy of ergotamine could be due to an effect on central nervous system serotoninergic neurons (Raskin 1981).

Let us for the moment presume that the vasoconstrictory effect of ergotamine is important for the therapeutic effect of ergotamine in migraine. How can we measure this effect? The measurements of temporal arterial pulsations, which would be a natural parameter, are difficult to interprete in physiological terms since they depend both on the blood is flow through the arteries, the stiffness of the arterial wall, and the real intra-arterial pulse pressure. Thus, injections of ergotamine and dihydroergotamine cause both decreases and increases of temporal arterial pulsations when used in the treatment of migraine attacks (Brazil and Friedman 1957). These measurements are therefore not suitable for pharmacological investigations.

In 1978 it was shown that ergotamine abusers with daily intake of ergotamine had subclinical ergotism as measured by strain gauge plethysmography (Dige-Petersen et al. 1977). Since then we have used this method to measure the effect of a single dose of ergotamine on extremity arteries. The strain gauge plethysmograph measures the systolic blood pressure (SBP) in, for example, a big toe. This SBP is extremely sensitive to constriction of the leg arteries, that is, that even a small constriction "so to say cuts off the tip of the pressure wave," leaving the diastolic blood pressure unchanged but significantly decreasing the SBP. What is measured with this method using suitable precautions (Tfelt-Hansen 1986) is thus a pure vasoconstrictory effect on arteries in man. The results are expressed as changes in systolic gradients, that is, toe SBP minus arm SBP (the arm SBP is used as a reference for systemic changes in blood pressure). A decrease in this systolic gradient thus means a constriction of the leg arteries. The main advantage of this indirect measurement of systolic gradients is that it is an atraumatic technqiue; thus measurements can be repeated, for example, up to 8 h with the equipment left untouched, which increases the reproduceability. Are these measurements on leg arteries relevant for the presumed effect of ergotamine on extracranial arteries? Probably, because ergotamine seems to act on a 5-HT receptor in both types of arteries (Müller-Schweinitzer and Weidman 1977).

Previously, ergotamine was characterized as a vasoconstrictor with a quickly reversible action (Rothlin and Cerletti 1949). The subclinical ergotism observed in ergotamine abusers (Dige-Petersen et al. 1977) could either be due to accumulation of ergotamine (or its effect) or to a long duration of a single dose of drug. We therefore investigated the duration of a single dose of ergotamine in migraine patients (Tfelt-Hansen et al. 1980). Seventeen patients received 0.5 mg ergotamine i.v. and ten patients received 2–4 mg ergotamine as suppositories. The results are shown in Figs. 4 and 5. Both a *single* i.v. and a rectal dose of ergotamine caused a decrease in toe-arm systolic gradients the day after administration. Ergotamine is therefore a *long-acting* arterial vasoconstrictor. In contrast, the effect on arterioles causes an increase in SBP lasting only 3 h (Tfelt-Hansen et al. 1980). Ergotamine therefore probably acts on arteries and arterioles by different mechanisms.

Next, we examined the responsiveness to ergotamine in ten former ergotamine abusers after 0.5 mg ergotamine i.v. (Tfelt-Hansen and Olesen 1981). The resulting decreases in ankle- and toe-arm systolic gradients were comparable to the decreases found in migraine patients who only occasionally used ergotamine (see Table 2). Furthermore, the decreases in ankle- and toe-arm systolic gradients observed during abuse of ergotamine suppositories (Dige-Petersen et al. 1977) are in the same range as found after a single rectal dose of ergotamine (Tfelt-Hansen

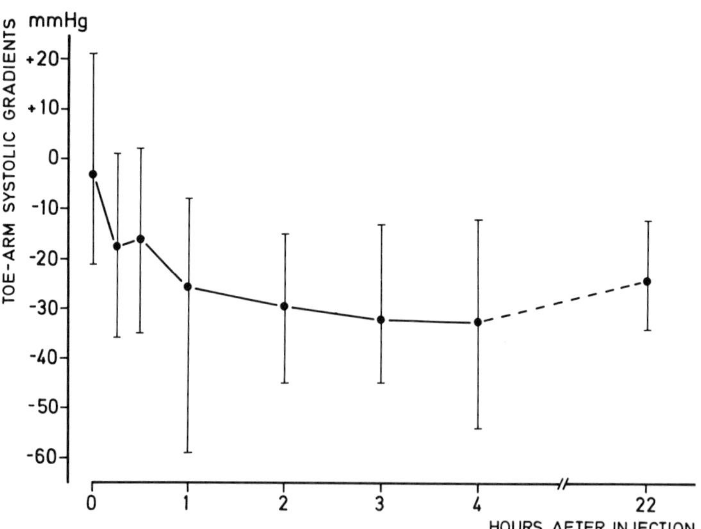

Fig. 4. The effect of 0.5 mg ergotamine tartrate i.v. on ten toe-arm systolic gradients in migraine patients. Note the slowly developing decrease in toe-arm systolic gradients, and that the effect was well sustained 22 h later. Means and ranges are given. (From Tfelt-Hansen 1986)

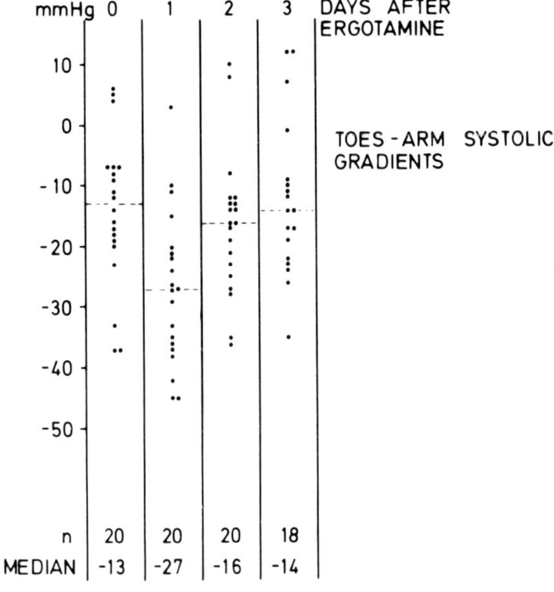

Fig. 5. Toe-arm systolic gradients after therapeutic rectal doses of ergotamine in migraine patients. Two patients received 4 mg and eight took 2 mg ergotamine tartrate as a suppository (*P* given for Wilcoxon's paired test). (From Tfelt-Hansen et al. 1980)

Table 2. Changes in toe- and ankle-arm systolic gradients in ten previously abusing and 17 nonabusing migraine patients.[a] (Data from Tfelt-Hansen and Olesen 1981)

	Abusers (mmHg)	Nonabusers (mmHg)
Maximum changes on day 1		
Toe-arm systolic gradient		
(Mean $\pm$ SD)	-27 ± 13	-29 ± 15
(Range)	$(-7 - -52)$	$(+1 - -56)$
Ankle-arm systolic gradient		
(Mean $\pm$ SD)	-15 ± 6	-15 ± 8
(Range)	$(-8 - -27)$	$(+5 - -36)$
Changes on day 2		
Toe-arm systolic gradient		
(Mean $\pm$ SD)	-14 ± 16	-18 ± 14
(Range)	$(+10 - -48)$	$(+8 - -47)$
Ankle-arm systolic gradient		
(Mean $\pm$ SD)	-10 ± 11	-13 ± 10
(Range)	$(+7 - -28)$	$(+7 - -31)$

[a] The two groups were comparable; $P > 0.05$ (Mann-Whitney rank sum test) for all parameters.

112   P. Tfelt-Hansen

et al. 1980). There are, therefore, no indications from these studies that hypersensitivity or tolerance to ergotamine develop during ergotamine abuse. The decreases in leg systolic gradients observed during abuse of ergotamine must be due to the long-lasting effect of the previous dose of ergotamine.

The effect of ergotamine on toe-arm systolic gradients is dose dependent (Tfelt-Hansen and Manniche 1984), and by measuring this parameter it could be shown that 1 mg ergotamine as a suppository is pharmacologically active, whereas no effect was found after 1 mg ergotamine orally (Bülow et al. 1986).

There is an apparent discrepancy between the time course for the kinetics of ergotamine (quickly distributed with a half-life of 3 min and quickly cleared with a biological half-life of 2 h, and the dynamic effect on arteries (slow onset and long duration of action) (Fig. 4). We analyzed this phenomenon by applying an "effect compartment model" to combine kinetic and dynamic data obtained in ten migraine patients (Tfelt-Hansen and Paalzow 1985). The basic assumption of the model is that the kinetics of the active site might not parallel the general kinetics of the drug. By applying this model one can obtain an estimate of the sensitivity of the subjects from nonequilibrium data: the plasma concentration which would cause 50% of a maximum effect in a hypothetical steady state ($Cp_{ss}50$) and an estimate of the rate constant at the active site (k_{eo}).

The mean plasma levels and mean decreases in toe-arm systolic gradients are shown in Fig. 6. The $Cp_{ss}50$ estimated from the mean data was 0.24 ng/ml. This plasma concentration is approximately 0.5×10^{-9} mol/liter, demonstrating that ergotamine is a very potent drug. The $Cp_{ss}50$ of 0.24 ng/ml is near the detection

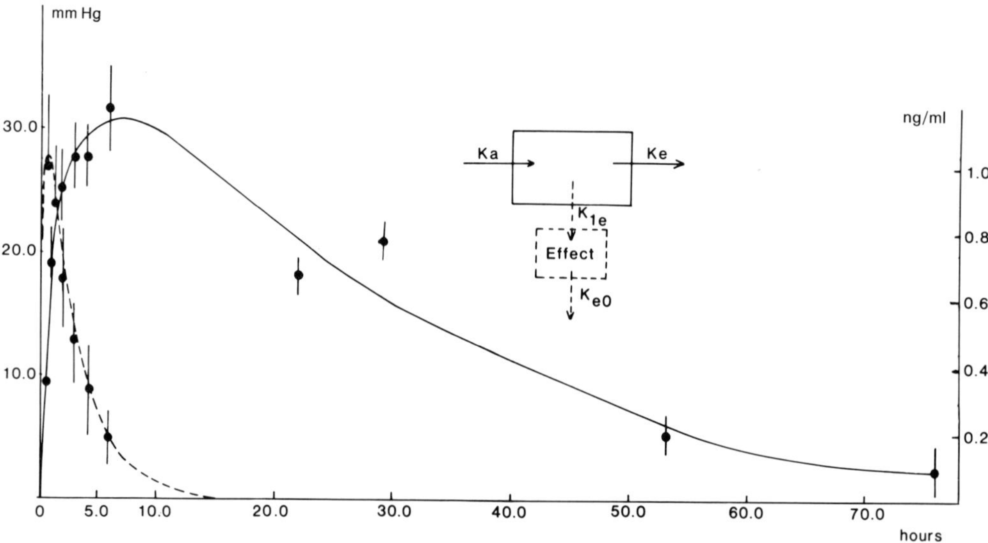

Fig. 6. Mean decrease in toe-arm systolic gradient and mean plasma concentration of ergotamine after 0.5 mg ergotamine tartrate i.m. to ten migraine patients. *Points* are actual measured values ($\pm$SEM) and *lines* show the computed fits. *Broken line*, plasma concentration of ergotamine (ng/ml); *solid line*, decrease in toe-arm systolic gradients (mmHg). The effect compartment is also shown. Note the huge discrepancy in time between the effect and the plasma levels. (From Tfelt-Hansen and Paalzow (1985)

Table 3. Effect model parameters for the effect of ergotamine on peripheral systolic blood pressure. For explanation see text. (Data from Tfelt-Hansen and Paalzow 1985)

Subject No.	k_{eo} (h^{-1})	$t_{\frac{1}{2}}k_{eo}$ (h)	$Cp_{ss}50$ (ng/ml)
1	0.074	9.37	0.508
2	0.015	46.21	0.078
3	0.058	11.95	1.787
4	0.082	8.45	0.792
5	0.078	8.89	0.128
6	0.064	10.83	0.829
7	0.073	9.49	0.065
8	0.022	30.9	0.044
9	0.070	9.86	0.059
10	0.038	18.24	1.443
$\bar{X}\pm$SD	0.057 ± 0.023	12.07 ± 5.04	0.573 ± 0.631
Calculated from mean data ($\pm$SD of parameters)	0.070 ± 0.004	9.90 ± 0.56	0.238 ± 0.029

limit of 0.1 ng/ml for the HPLC method (Edlund 1981). It can be estimated that if steady state concentrations of 0.1 ng/ml, 0.05 ng/ml, and 0.025 ng/ml were reached, this would result in decreases of the toe-arm systolic gradients of 25, 18, and 12 mmHg, respectively (Tfelt-Hansen 1986). These estimates might explain why we can observe an effect of ergotamine despite almost unmeasurable plasma levels with the HPLC method after rectal administration of ergotamine (Tfelt-Hansen et al. 1980). From the calculations using mean data the k_{eo} was found to be 0.07 h^{-1}. Ergotamine is thus very slowly dissociated from the active site with a half-life of 10 h.

The model was also used to estimate individual $Cp_{ss}50$ and k_{eo} for each patient, as shown in Table 3. The greatest interindividual variability was found for the sensitivity parameter $Cp_{ss}50$. This large variability reflects both the error in measuring the effect and in modelling, and the interindividual variability in sensitivity to ergotamine. Thus, the variability in sensitivity is probably overestimated. Interindividual differences in reaction to ergotamine were, however, found in a dose-response study (Tfelt-Hansen and Manniche 1984), and it is my qualified guess that migraine patients vary with a factor of 10 in their sensitivity to ergotamine.

We have recently studied the effect of ergotamine and dihydroergotamine on cerebral blood flow (CBF) in man (Andersen et al. 1987). It was previously shown that i.m. ergotamine did not decrease CBF measured after 15–20 min (Hachinsky et al. 1978). As mentioned above, the arterial vasoconstrictory effect of ergotamine is, however, not maximal until after 4–6 h. We therefore measured the effect of 0.5 mg ergotamine i.v. and 1 mg dihydroergotamine i.v. after 4 h. Both the resting CBF and CBF increased by acetazolamide were unchanged in eight normal male volunteers (non-migraine sufferers).

Some Clinical Implications

Ergotamine is a drug with a very low rectal bioavailability and an extremely low oral bioavailability (Ibraheem et al. 1983). The addition of possible active metabolites can be judged from the extent to which they are formed into other ergotalkaloids.

Seven- to ten-fold higher concentrations for active metabolites than for the parent substance (Maurer and Frick 1984; Bredberg et al. 1986) result in only a few percent "total oral bioavailability" which is still very low.

The problem is, however, not that the bioavailability is low but that it – as with other drugs with a low bioavailability – is very variable. There is thus a considerable *kinetic variability* among patients. Furthermore, added to the kinetic variability, a *dynamic variability* – interindividual differences in sensitivity (Tfelt-Hansen and Paalzow 1985) – should be anticipated. There can, therefore, be no standard dose of the drug when used orally or rectally, but the dose should be tailored to the individual patient by trial and error. What dose should then be the starting dose in this process? Since we have shown that 1 mg ergotamine is pharmacologically active rectally (Bülow et al. 1986), we suggest that this should be the starting dose.

Apart from the acute side effects of ergotamine, which deter some patients from using the drug, the major medical problem with this drug is, of course, *ergotamine abuse*. We have shown that previous ergotamine abusers have the same sensitivity to ergotamine as other migraine patients (Tfelt-Hansen and Olesen 1981). Thus the abuse is not due to hypersensitivity or tolerance to the drug. In order to avoid the chronic vasoconstriction which is the most probable cause of the symptoms and the withdrawal headache, it is important to be aware that the *duration of effect of a single dose* of ergotamine is 24 h. Thus, the interval between each dose of ergotamine should be at least 48 h.

Finally, can ergotamine – a vasoconstrictor – be used in classic migraine where there is probably ischemia during the aura phase? Our studies as well as those of other authors have so far not shown any effect of ergotamine on CBF in normal man (Andersen et al. 1987; Hachinsky et al. 1978). Migraine patients might have a different cerebrovascular reactivity, and until the effect of ergotamine on CBF in migraine patients has been studied further, I would not recommend the use of ergotamine in patients with prolonged (> 30 min) aura symptoms.

References

Aellig WH (1984) Investigation of the venoconstrictor effect of 8′hydroxydihydroergotamine, the main metabolite of dihydroergotamine, in man. Eur J Clin Pharmacol 26:239–242

Aellig WH, Nüesch E (1977) Comparative pharmacokinetic investigations with tritium-labelled ergot alkaloids after oral and intravenous administration in man. Int J Clin Pharmacol 15:106–112

Ala-Hurula V, Myllylä VV, Arvela P, Heikkilä J, Kärki N, Hokannen E (1979 a) Systemic availability of ergotamine tartrate after oral, rectal and intramuscular administration. Eur J Clin Pharmacol 15:51–55

Ala-Hurula V, Myllylä VV, Arvela P, Kärki N, Hokkanen E (1979 b) Systemic availability of ergotamine tartrate after three successive doses and during continuous medication. Eur J Clin Pharmacol 16:355–360

Andersen AR, Tfelt-Hansen P, Lassen NA (1987) The effect of ergotamine and dihydroergotamine on cerebral blood flow in man. Stroke 18:120–123

Andersson PG (1975) Ergotamine headache. Headache 15:118–121

Brazil P, Friedman AP (1957) Further observations in craniovascular studies. Neurology 7:52–55

Bredberg U, Eyjolfsdottier GS, Paalzow L, Tfelt-Hansen P, Tfelt-Hansen V (1986) Pharmakokinetics of methysergide and its metabolite methylergometrine in man. Eur J Clin Pharmacol 30:75–77

Bülow PM, Ibraheem JJ, Paalzow G, Tfelt-Hansen P (1986) Comparison of pharmacodynamic effects and plasma levels of oral and rectal ergotamine. Cephalalgia 6:107–111

Dige-Petersen H, Lassen NA, Noer I, Tønnesen KH, Olesen J (1977) Subclinical ergotism. Lancet 2:65–66

Edlung P-O (1981) Determination of ergot alkaloids in plasma by high performance liquid chromatography and fluorescence detection. J Chromatogr 226:107–115

Ekbom K, Krabbe A, Paalzow G, Paalzow L, Tfelt-Hansen P, Waldenlind E (1983) Optimal routes of administration of ergotamine tartrate in cluster headache patients. A pharmacokinetic study. Cephalalgia 3:15–20

Graham JR, Wolff HG (1938) Mechanism of migraine headache and action of ergotamine tartrate. Arch Neurol Psychiatr 39:737–763

Hachinsky W, Norris JW, Edmeads J, Cooper PW (1978) Ergotamine and cerebral blood flow. Stroke 9:594–596

Haering N, Settlage JA, Sanders SW, Schuberth R (1985) Measurement of ergotamine in human plasma by triple sector quadrupole mass spectrometry with negative chemical ionization. Biomed Mass Spectrom 12:197–199

Hakkarainen H, Vapaatalo H, Gothoni G, Parantainen J (1979) Tolfenamic acid is as effective as ergotamine during migraine attacks. Lancet II:326–328

Ibraheem JJ, Paalzow L, Tfelt-Hansen P (1982) Kinetics of ergotamine after intravenous and intramuscular administration to migraine sufferers. Eur J Clin Pharmacol 23:235–240

Ibraheem JJ, Paalzow L, Tfelt-Hansen P (1983) Low bioavailability of ergotamine tartrate after oral and rectal administration in migraine sufferers. Br J Clin Pharmacol 16:695–699

Ibraheem JJ, Paalzow L, Tfelt-Hansen P (1985) Linear kinetics of intravenous ergotamine tartrate. Eur J Clin Pharmacol 29:61–66

Maurer G, Frick W (1984) Elucidation of the structure and receptor binding studies of the major primary metabolite of dihydroergotamine in man. Eur J Clin Pharmacol 26:463–470

Müller-Schweinitzer E, Weidman H (1977) Regional differences in the responsiveness of isolated arteries from cattle, dog and man. Agents Actions 7:383–389

Rall TW, Schleifer LS (1980) In: Gilman AG, Goodman LS, Gilman A (eds) The pharmacological basis of therapeutics, 6th edn. Macmillan, New York, p 946

Raskin NH (1981) Pharmacology of migraine. Annu Rev Pharmacol Toxicol 21:463–478

Rosenthaler J, Munzer H, Voges R, Andres H, GUll P, Bolliger G (1984) Immunoassay of ergotamine and dihydroergotamine using a common ^{3}H-labelled ligand as tracer for specific antibody and means to overcome experienced pitfalls. Int J Nucl Med Biol 11:85–89

Rothlin E, Cerletti E (1949) Untersuchungen über die Kreislaufwirkungen des Ergotamins. Helv Physiol Acta 7:333–370

Rowsell AR, Neylan C, Wilkinson M (1973) Ergotamine induced headache in migrainous patients. Headache 13:65–67

Sanders SW, Haering N, Mosberg H, Jaeger H (1986) Pharmacokinetics of ergotamine in healthy volunteers following oral and rectal dosing. Eur J Clin Pharmacol 30:331–334

Schlientz W, Brunner R, Hofman A, Berde B, Stürmer E (1961) Umlagerung von Mutterkornalkaloid-Präparaten in schwach sauren Lösungen. Pharmakologische Wirkungen der Isomerisierungsprodukte. Pharm Acta Helv 36:472–488

Tfelt-Hansen P (1986) The effect of ergotamine on the arterial system in man. Acta Pharmacol Toxicol (Copenh) 59[Suppl]3:1–30

Tfelt-Hansen P, Manniche PM (1984) Dose-response curve for the ergotamine-induced decrease of peripheral systolic blood pressure in man. Acta Pharmacol Toxicol (Copenh) 55:238–241

Tfelt-Hansen P, Olesen J (1981) Arterial response to ergotamine tartrate in abusing and non-abusing migraine patients. Acta Pharmacol Toxicol (Copenh) 48:69–72

Tfelt-Hansen P, Paalzow L (1985) Intramuscular ergotamine: plasma levels and dynamic activity. Clin Pharmacol Ther 37:29–35

Tfelt-Hansen P, Eickhoff JH, Olesen J (1980) The effect of single dose ergotamine tartrate on peripheral arteries in migraine patients: methodological aspects and time effect curve. Acta Pharmacol Toxicol (Copenh) 47:151–156

Tfelt-Hansen P, Jansen I, Edvinson L (1987) Methylergometrine antagonizes 5HT in the temporal artery. Eur J Clin Pharmacol 33:77–79

Ergotamine Tartrate Dependency: Possible Mechanisms

J. R. SAPER

For over 50 years, ergotamine tartrate (ET) has been considered the drug of first choice for an acute attack of migraine. Estimated effectiveness occurs in up to 90% of instances when the drug is used parenterally, 80% rectally, and in 50% orally (Dalessio 1980). ET has a stimulating effect on smooth muscle which produces vasoconstriction, an effect on medullary tissues causing a sympatholytic reaction, and a peripheral alpha-adrenergic blocking action (Rall and Schleifer 1980). Although assumed historically to be related to vasoconstriction, the specific influence of ET on migraine is not known with absolute certainty. Early reports by Dalessio et al. (1961) and more recent work by this author (Saper and van Meter 1980; Saper 1983; Saper and Jones 1986) have raised the possibility that the mechanism by which ergot derivatives affect migraine may be by both central as well as peripheral effects.

The common, untoward reactions of ET usage are well known and include nausea, vomiting, muscle achiness, diarrhea, and difficulty in swallowing. Ergotism, a more serious consequence of ergot therapy, is well delineated by Andersson (in this volume). Although usually the result of excessive dosage, serious reactions have been recorded at acceptable treatment levels or when the drug is taken in the presence of contraindications, such as peripheral vascular disease, hypertension, and ischemic heart disease (Saper 1983; Enge and Silvertssen 1965).

This chapter will draw attention to what appears to be a common (Saper and Jones 1986) but infrequently noted (Wolfson and Graham 1949; Friedman et al. 1955; Horton and Peters 1963; Tfelt-Hansen and Krabbe 1981) and previously poorly understood condition, that of ergotamine dependency and its clinical consequences. Occassionally referred to as "ergot headache" or "rebound headache", (Lippman 1955; Rowsell et al. 1973; Anderson 1975; Ala-Hurula et al. 1982) the hallmark of this condition is a self-sustaining, rhythmic headache/medication cycle, characterized by daily or almost daily migraine headaches and an irresistible and predictable use of ergotamine tartrate as the only means of alleviating the headache attacks. When present, the syndrome appears to render all other appropriate treatments relatively ineffective. If left untreated, this condition may serve as the forerunner of frank ergotism.

Michigan Headache and Neurological Institute, 3120, Professional Drive, Ann Arbor, MI 48104, USA

Drug-Induced Headache
Ed. by H.-C. Diener and M. Wilkinson
© Springer-Verlag Berlin Heidelberg 1988

Background

Lippman (1955) described a characteristic headache resulting from prolonged use of ergot derivatives calling the phenomenon the "ergotamine headache". The headache was described as a dull, daily, and usually constant head pain. Acute migraine would result if ergotamine was withheld. Ironically, despite the apparent widespread nature of this problem, relatively few subsequent reports have specifically adressed this problem (Rowsell et al. 1973; Andersson 1975; Saper and van Meter 1980; Tfelt-Hansen and Krabbe 1981; Ala-Hurula et al. 1982).

In a report to the American Association for the Study of Headache (Saper and van Meter 1980) we described 32 patients with intractable daily headaches whose history reflected the daily or almost daily use of ET as the only means of pain alleviation and referred to this condition as "ergotamine habituation." These 32 patients, together with many others presented and hundreds of others with this disorder whom we have encountered in practice, prompt our belief that sufficient support exists to satisfy criteria establishing a physical state of dependency in some patients using ET excessively.

The Existence of a State of Dependency

"Physical dependence" (habituation) is defined as the continued use of a drug, the deprivation of which gives rise to symptoms of distress, abstinence, and withdrawal, and accompanied by an irresistible impulse to take the drug. In order to establish successfully that such a condition exists, the following three conditions must be met:

1. Documentation of a predictable and irresistible pattern of usage
2. The development of tolerance
3. A state of abstinence or withdrawal upon discontinuance of medication

In a work previously published (Saper and Jones 1986) we detailed the evidence in support of the state of dependency for ET. This argument will not be repeated in detail here, but a summary of that argument follows. After a review of the many case reports including reports of other authors as well as our own work (Wolfson and Graham 1949; Friedman et al. 1955; Lippman 1955; Horton and Peters 1963; Rowsell et al. 1973; Anderson 1975; Tfelt-Hansen and Krabbe 1981; Ala-Hurula et al. 1982; Saper and Jones 1986; Saper, to be published), it appears that all well-described cases reflect a predictable headache/medication cycle occurring with a background of daily or almost daily usage. All case reports further describe the reliable effectiveness of ET which is characteristically the only means of headache relief. Moreover, the frequency of usage exceeds natural frequency of migraine (Ad Hoc Committee on Classification of Headache 1962; World Federation of Neurology 1969; Lance 1982). Migraine is a variable disorder with an irregular pattern of occurrence which may vary from week to week and month to month. Rarely does migraine, in its natural state, occur more than once or twice a week and usually considerably less often. In the cases reported, an unnatural frequency of vascular headache occurs daily or almost daily. And, because ET is specific for vascular headache, and because the headache patterns are both migraine like and characteristically responsive to ET, it is concluded that migraine occurs at an unnatural frequency and in response to ET.

Case reports clearly demonstrate an increasing pattern of usage and total weekly dosage. Despite daily or weekly dosage totals which frequently exceed safety limitations, patients demonstrate few serious consequences and thus fulfill the definition of tolerance. Of the 32 patients in our 1980 report, 12 were taking more than 10 mg ET per week, 12 were taking more than 15 mg per week, and six were taking more than 26 mg per week. In our 1986 report (Saper and Jones 1986) three patients exceeded 10 mg per week, and in one case 10–15 mg ET were required daily. In a current report in preparation (Saper, to be published), three new patients demonstrated a daily usage pattern of 6 mg or more per day and a weekly dose that exceeded 40 mg per week. Nonetheless, only one patient in the 1980 report and none of the other cases reported demonstrated evidence of clinically identifiable or significant peripheral ischemia.

Upon discontinuance of the drug, a predictable and definable protracted and severely debilitating headache episode occurs, accompanied by autonomic disturbances and other somatic and mental complaints fulfilling the definition of "abstinence" (Saper and van Meter 1980; Ala-Hurula et al. 1982; Saper and Jones 1986). This prolonged attack usually occurs within 72 h following withholding of the drug and may last 72 h and longer once it begins. Moreover, a review of our data from our 1980 study (Saper and van Meter 1980) suggested that no discernible differences could be detected in the patterns of headache or in other events following discontinuance when comparing patients using ET preparations containing caffeine or barbiturates and those whose preparations contained ET alone. Upon discontinuance, patients either improved spontaneously without additional treatment (Tfelt-Hansen and Krabbe 1981) or improved with preventative treatment programs which had been largely without benefit earlier (Saper and van Meter 1980; Saper and Jones 1986; Saper, to be published). In the excellent work of Tfelt-Hansen and Krabbe (1981), 40 patients using ET frequently demonstrated improvement in overall headache control upon discontinuance and without the administration of preventative treatment. According to this report, discontinuance represented the critical factor in reducing headache frequency. In the cases reported in our 1986 (Saper and Jones 1986) and 1980 (Saper and van Meter 1980) reports, all patients also improved clinically following ET discontinuance, and in most of these cases the prophylactic treatments had been of no value prior to ET discontinuance.

Clinical Features and Recognition

The characteristic clinical features of this syndrome are the following. Headache of a migraine type occurs on a daily or almost daily basis. As the effects of the previous dose of ET wane, the headache typically escalates until the next dose of ET is administered. Psychological dependency intensifies, and depression and sleep disturbance are frequently noted. Whether the latter symptoms are the direct result of the drug on central (brain) mechanisms (see below) or on other factors is undetermined. The headache is strikingly sensitive to ET but will not generally respond to alternate symptomatic or preventative medications which would otherwise be expected to have an ameliorating effect.

Because migraine rarely occurs more than once or twice a week and is characteristically a variable disorder, a migraine headache occurring more than two or three times a week and which is selectively responsive to ET while refractory to other symptomatic or preventative medications should serve to alert to the possible presence of this disorder.

Typically, patients will report an increasing frequency of headaches and will request larger supplies of ET. Traditional restrictions and warning on the use of ET have been based on the *total dosage per week*, not frequency of use. Thus, patient requests for more medicine may not seem particularly troublesome initially since total weekly dose limits may not be exceeded in a patient taking up to 10 mg to 14 mg per week – 1–2 mg a day, 5–7 days per week. Reported cases (Saper and van Meter 1980; Saper and Jones 1986) document that patients taking as little as ½–1 mg three or four times per week may be affected by this syndrome, although most patients demonstrate greater dosages and frequency.

From patient surveys, it appears that increasing usage results from either patient-determined preventative administration for "expected" but not yet present migraine attacks or from attempts to treat nonmigrainous tension or daily chronic headache with ET. Patients also cite the advice of their physicians to take ET as early as possible in the course of a headache, thus prompting usage before the exact nature of a headache or its full manifestations become apparent. Patients confirm their use of ET at the first sign of any headache (many have nonmigrainous forms, Saper 1986) or when experiencing some vague, abnormal sense that they believe *might* represent a *pre*-headache prodrome.

Mechanism of Dependency: A Hypothesis

The exact mechanism of ergot dependency is unknown. However, it is proposed that it is related to the central (brain) influences and the metabolic nature of this substance (Saper and Jones 1986). Accumulation and storage of ET in body tissue occur after a single administration, and a secondary blood level peak at least 12 h after an administration has been demonstrated (Ala-Hurula et al. 1979a, b). Although the half-life of ET is 95 ± 30 min, a slow elimination half-life of 34 h has been shown (Wilkinson and Orton 1980). The slow elimination might explain the clinical phenomena in those who appear to have used the drug every 2nd or 3rd day rather than daily.

Of possible importance is the poor systemic availability of ET in patients who overuse it. A good correlation between symptoms following discontinuance and plasma levels is lacking (Ala-Hurula et al. 1979a, b, 1982; Ekbom et al. 1981; Hovdal et al. 1982). CSF levels have been detected and do correlate with the plasma levels in one report (Ala-Hurula et al. 1979b), but not in another (Hovdal et al. 1982), suggesting that crossing of the blood-brain barrier is likely and of possible importance.

While studying the characteristics of chronic daily headache (Saper et al. 1983), we noted that patients using daily or excessive amounts of ET were more likely to exhibit positive dexamethasone suppression tests (DST) than headache patients taking daily analgesics. The DST reflects neuroendocrine function of the limbic-hypothalamic-pituitary-adrenal (LHPA) axis and is used in the assessment of melancholia (Carroll et al. 1981). In further studies on the mechanism and clinical implications of ergotamine dependency, we evaluated the DST in 40 patients in a combined retrospective and prospective study (Saper and Jones 1985). These patients were compared with 40 controls, matched as closely as possible for age and sex. The results of our study demonstrate a positive test in 65% of cases (ergot users) compared to 27.5% of controls, representing a more than twofold increase, with a $\chi^2 = 11.32$ ($P < 0.001$). The cortisol level compared between groups demonstrated a mean value of 15.6 mg/dl for test patients (ergot users) compared with a mean of 5.24 mg/dl for controls, a three-fold difference with a $T_{78} = 3.39$ ($P < 0.005$). In addition, although the number of patients at higher dosages was small, a trend toward a direct relationship between cortisol secretion (failure to suppress) and a greater ergotamine dosage was noted.

It is known that LHPA regulation involves corticotropin-releasing factor, adrenocorticotropic hormone, cortisol, catecholamines, indolamines, and gamma-aminobutyric acid. It is also known that ET increases turnover and inhibits norepinephrine synthesis, which in turn increases cortisol secretion. Ergot also acts as a noncompetitive inhibitor of 5-hydroxytryptamine (serotonin) which also increases cortisol secretion (Fuxe et al. 1978; Lemburger 1978; Silbergeld and Hruska 1979; Saper 1986). It is proposed that the influence of ET in altering the results of the DST might reflect its effect on biogenic amines or aminergic receptors which in turn control the rhythmic secretion of cortisol. The LHPA which thus appears influenced by ET usage is also the purported locus for migraine accompaniments such as depression, sleep disturbance, emotional lability, appetite disturbances, hormone regulation, and emotions.

The upper brainstem and the LHPA are also considered important in the proposed central mechanism of migraine (Lance 1982, 1987). Lance (1982) has shown that stimulation of the locus ceruleus in the pons results in the neurovascular changes recognized to occur during migraine. The locus ceruleus is mediated by norepinephrine, and it is possible that frequent or daily use of ET might alter the sensitivity of the neurotransmitter or receptor function in these areas, resulting in "rebound" or "reflex hyperactivity" following discontinuance and/or reduction in blood drug levels following last usage. The abstinence phenomena (rebound) due to ET could thus be similar to the abstinence syndromes of opiate, nicotine, and alcohol, all of which are thought to be related to disturbances in the locus ceruleus (Gold et al. 1980; Bakris et al. 1982; Glassman and Jackson 1984). In essence, the neurovascular changes of rebound might in part reflect overreactivity of the locus ceruleus, the cells of which are noradrenergic.

In addition to the above, a chronobiological factor may be very important in the mechanism of ergotamine dependency. Through its influence on serotonin and norepinephrine receptors in the brainstem and/or through an ascending in-

fluence via the dorsal raphe nucleus on the hypothalamic pacemaker (suprachias-
mic nuclei), it is possible that ET exerts an important physiological influence on
circadian or other hypothalamic rhythms. The circadian rhythm of serotonin,
which peaks during the day and falls during the night, may actually be "captured"
by a synchronizing influence of daily ET. The strong relevance of serotonin to the
proposed mechanisms of migraine and to the ascending influence on the hypo-
thalamus may well play an important and critical role in the dependency/addic-
tion process.

The order and process by which this phenomenon occurs is not yet known.
Whether the primary factor begins as a natural increase in the frequency of headache, followed by the increased use of ET and eventually the dependency phenomena or, on the other hand, whether increasingly frequent use of ET, perhaps
by its prophylactic administration, induces more headaches is yet uncertain.
Moreover, whether the accompanying depression and sleep disturbance are
simply natural components of recurring headache or the result of the central effects of ET remains speculative. Many patients who are interviewed regarding
their increasing usage suggest that an increasing nonmigrainous headache may
have, in retrospect, prompted the increasing use of ET.

Treatment and Prevention

The treatment of this condition begins with the withdrawal of all ET. Hospitalization is frequently advised during which supportive measures are instituted including i.v. fluids to control fluid and electrolyte changes when nausea and vomiting are present. Symptomatic narcotic and phenothiazine administration, usually
via parenteral routes, is employed when necessary. In our hospital headache unit
(Saper and van Meter 1981; van Meter and Saper 1983) we have recently employed a variation of the Raskin protocol (Raskin 1986) for i.v. dihydroergotamine (DHE) therapy during the initial phases of ergotamine withdrawal. This
enhances patient compliance and assists in a gradual reduction of ergot derivatives. We have also employed clonidine hydrochloride to control abstinence phenomena. A well-trained team of supportive and experienced professionals who
employ appropriate treatment protocols to assist patients through the very painful days during the initial process of hospitalization is worthwhile. After withdrawal, patients may notice a spontaneous and dramatic reduction in headache
intensity and frequency, even without prophylactic agents. For those that require
preventative therapy, prophylaxis with beta-adrenergic blocking agents and/or a
tricyclic antidepressant is frequently effective. Symptomatic headache control can
be achieved with Midrin, analgesics, or even occasionally ET, provided the use
of ET does not exceed more than a couple of administrations per month.

It is clear from the experience of this author that ET can evolve with a background of increasing ET usage that exceeds a frequency of greater than two dosage days per week. Patients must be limited to this maximum frequency. Prophylactic agents must be employed with appropriate intensity in order to maintain
this control. Careful monitoring of drug usage patterns and limited amounts of
drug per prescription are strongly advised.

Conclusion

The frequent use of ET can result in a state of psychological and physiological dependency which promotes increasing usage of the drug and daily or almost daily headaches of a migraine type. The early onset of this condition is insidious and may result from either too frequent administrations of the drug for nonmigrainous forms of headache or from self-initiated prophylactic usage. The actual mechanism appears to involve central disturbances involving hypothalamic and brainstem mechanisms. The syndrome can be prevented by limiting the use of ET to no more than 2 dosage days per week. Once withdrawal occurs in those patients who go through abstinence, the pre-existent headache disturbance re-emerges, often with a dramatic lessening of migraine frequency (with or without treatment).

References

Ad Hoc Committee (1962) Classification of Headache. JAMA 179:717–718

Ala-Hurula V, Myllya VV, Arvela P et al. (1979 a) Systemic availability of ergotamine tartrate after oral, rectal, and intramuscular administration. Eur J Clin Pharmacol 15:51–55

Ala-Hurula V, Myllya VV, Arvela P et al. (1979 b) Systemic availability of ergotamine tartrate after three successive dosages during continuous medication. Eur J Clin Pharmacol 16:355–360

Ala-Hurula V, Myllyla VV, Hokkanen E (1982) Ergotamine buse: results of ergotamine discontinuance with special reference to plasma concentrations. Cephalgia 2:189–195

Andersson PG (1975) Ergotamine headache. Headache 15:118–121

Bakris GL, Cross PD, Hammarstein JE (1982) The use of clonidine for management of opiate abstinence in a chronic pain patient. Mayo Clin Proc 57:657–660

Carroll BJ, Feinberg M, Greden JF et al. (1981) A specific laboratory test for the diagnosis of melancholia. Arch Gen Psychiatry 1981; 38:15–22

Dalessio DJ (1980) Wolff's headaches and other pain (4th edn). Oxford University Press, New York

Dalessio DJ, Camp WA, Goodell H, Wolff HG (1961) Studies on headache. The mode of action of UML-491 in its relevance to the nature of vascular headache of the migraine type. Arch Neurol 4:235

Ekbom K, Paalzow L, Waldenlind E (1981) Low biological availability of ergotamine tartrate after dosing in cluster headache. Cephalgia 1:203–207

Enge I, Silvertssen E (1965) Ergotism due to therapeutic doses of ergotamine tartrate. Am Heart J 70:665–670

Friedman AP, Brazil P, von Storch TJC (1955) Ergotamine tolerance in patients with migraine. JAMA 157:881–884

Fuxe K, Fredholm BB, Ogren S et al. (1978) Ergot drugs and central monoaminergic mechanisms: a histochemical, biochemical, and behavioral analysis. Fed Proc 37:2181–2191

Glassman AH, Jackson WK (1984) Cigarette craving, smoking withdrawal and clonidine. Science 226:864

Gold MS, Pottash AC, Sweeny DR et al. (1980) Opiate withdrawal using clonidine, a safe, effective, and rapid non-opiate treatment. JAMA 243:343–346

Horton BT, Peters GA (1963) Clinical manifestations of excessive use of ergotamine preparations and manifestations of withdrawal effect. Report of 52 cases. Headache 2:214–227

Hovdal H, Syversen GB, Rosenthaler J (1982) Ergotamine in plasma and CSF after IM and rectal administration to humans. Cephalgia 2:145–150

Lance JW (1982) Mechanisms in management of headache (4th edn). Butterworth: Boston

Lance JW (1987) Pathogenesis of migraine. In: Saper JR (ed) Controversies and clinical variants of migraine. Pergamon, New York

Lemburger L (1978) The pharmacology of ergots: past and present. Fed Proc (1955) 37:2176–2180

Lippman CW (1955) Characteristic headache resulting from prolonged use of ergot derivatives. J Nerv Men Dis 121:270–273

Rall TW, Schleifer LS (1980) Drugs affecting uterine motility. In: Goodman LS, Wilman A (eds) The physiological basis of therapeutics (6th edn) Mac Millan, New York, pp 935–950

Raskin NH (1986) Repetitive intravenous dihydroergotamine as therapy for intractable migraine. Neurology 36:995–997

Rowsell AR, Neylan C, Wilkinson M (1973) Ergotamine induced headache in migraine patients. Headache 13:65–67

Saper J (1983) Headache disorders: current concepts and treatment strategies. Wright-PSG, Littleton MA

Saper JR (1986) Changing perspectives on chronic headache. Clin J Pain 2:19–28

Saper JR, Jones JM (1985) Hypothalamic-pituitary-adrenal (HPA) disturbances in ergotamine "rebound" headache: clinical and mechanistic implications (Abstr). Headache 25:163–164

Saper JR, Jones JM (1986) Ergotamine dependency. Clin Neuropharmacol 9:244–256

Saper JR, Van Meter MJ (1980) Ergotamine habituation: analysis and profile (Abstr). Headache 20:159

Saper JR, Van Meter MJ (1981) An inpatient headache unit: development, directives, and struggles (Abstr). Headache 2:126

Saper JR, Johnson T, Van Meter M (1983) Mixed headache: a chronic headache process – a study of 500 patients (Abstr). Headache 23:143

Silbergeld EK, Hruska RE (1979) Effects of ergot drugs on serotonergic function: behavior and neurochemistry. Eur J Pharmacol 58:1–10

Tfelt-Hansen P, Krabbe AA (1981) Ergotamine abuse. Do patients benefit from withdrawal? Cephalgia 1:29–32

Van Meter Mj, Saper JR (1983) Inpatient treatment of intractable headache – an outcome study. Headache 23:144

Wilkinson M, Orton D (1980) Some observations on the use of ergotamine tartrate. Headache 20:159

Wolfson WQ, Graham JR (1949) Development of tolerance to ergot alkaloids in a patient with unusually severe migraine. N Engl J Med 241:296–298

World Federation of Neurology (1969) J Neurol Sci 9:202

Platelet Reactivity in Ergotamine Headache Compared to Migraine and Muscle Contraction Headache

K.-H. Grotemeyer, H.-P. Schlake, and I. W. Husstedt

Introduction

Enhanced platelet reactivity in migraine seems well established (Grotemeyer et al. 1983; Lechner et al. 1985). The basis for the observed change in platelet function is still unknown (Kruglak et al. 1984). Abnormal platelet reactivity could represent a side effect of migraine (Deshmuk and Meyer 1977), it could be a pure epiphenomenon (Rose 1985), or it may be an important step in the evolution of a migraine headache (Hannington et al. 1981).

Ergotamine headache shows a clinical picture which is in some respects similar to migraine headache. Most patients suffer from ergotamine headache because they are not able to distinguish migraine from ergotamine headache and therefore take even more ergotamine. The purpose of these study is to determine platelet function in ergotamine headache and to compare these findings with those obtained in migraine and muscle contraction headache.

Methods

Platelet activating time is only 100 ms (Born 1982). This finding indicates that there is no way of obtaining a blood sample without activating platelets by blood sampling. The platelet reactivity test (PR) as described earlier (Grotemeyer and Hofferberth 1985) was introduced to determine the activation of platelet function induced by blood sampling. In general 300 µl blood were suspended both in ethylenediaminotetraacetate (EDTA) and in EDTA-formaldehyde. Red blood cells were counted in both samples. The platelets activated and aggregated by blood collection were dissolved in EDTA and fixed in EDTA-formaldehyde. By centrifugation, aggregates sink to the bottom and are not present in the supernatant fluid while single platelets remain in the supernatant fluid. The PR increases proportionately with the number of platelet aggregates.

$$\frac{\text{EDTA platelets} \times \text{EDTA formaldehyde-erythrocytes}}{\text{EDTA formaldehyde-platelets} \times \text{EDTA erythrocytes}}$$

The test system was standardized in 110 healthy persons (50 women, 60 men, age 48 ± 16 years).

Department of Neurology, University of Münster, Albert-Schweitzer-Str. 33, D-4400 Münster, Federal Republic of Germany

Drug-Induced Headache
Ed. by H.-C. Diener and M. Wilkinson
© Springer-Verlag Berlin Heidelberg 1988

Headache Classification

This study includes 147 patients examined in the headache ward of the Department of Neurology; for the classification of headache the following criteria were employed:

- Common migraine was diagnosed according to the Ad Hoc Committee on Classification of Headache (1962), but only when attacks were not more frequent than six per month and the attacks were accompanied by nausea and/or vomiting at the start of the attack.
- Muscle contraction headache (MCH) was diagnosed when headache started in the neck and went to the forehead and persisted inconstantly for hours, days, or weeks. Vomiting after a fully developed headache was in agreement with the diagnosis. The sternocleidomastoid muscles were painful at the mastoid insertion in all cases.
- Ergotamine headache was diagnosed when a "typical" migraine attack occurred three or more times a week with a good response to ergotamine tartrate application.

Patients

A total of 85 patients suffering from common migraine were investigated, 70 women and 15 men, age 34 ± 12 years. In addition 30 patients (20 women, 10 men, age 38 ± 15 years) with MCH were included in the study. Finally PR was calculated in 32 patients with the diagnosis of ergotamine headache (24 women, eight men, age 40 ± 15 years). Regular ergotamine medication had been taken from 7 months to 15 years. Headache frequency was three to six times a week. Ergotamine dosage ranged from 2.25–21 mg/per week. All patients were tested when they had been headache free for at least 12 h. Intake of acetylsalicylic acid was excluded in all cases.

Results

PR in healthy persons was 0.98 ± 0.09. No sex or age influence could be observed. Platelet reactivity in migraine patients was 1.34 ± 0.31 on average. In MCH patients PR was 1.04 ± 0.18 (Fig. 1). In patients suffering from ergotamine headache PR was 1.20 ± 0.16 (Fig. 2). Differences between healthy persons and migraine or ergotamine headache patients were significant ($P < 0.01$). MCH patients and healthy persons showed no significant differences.

Re-examination 8 weeks after ergotamine withdrawal allowed a definitive classification of headache in 28 patients. Ten patients were identified as suffering from MCH and 18 patients showed typical common migraine headache. In four patients it was impossible to classify headache. PR in ten patients with MCH was

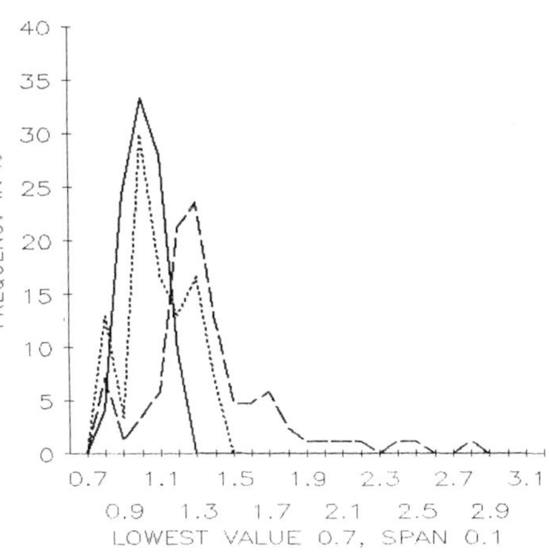
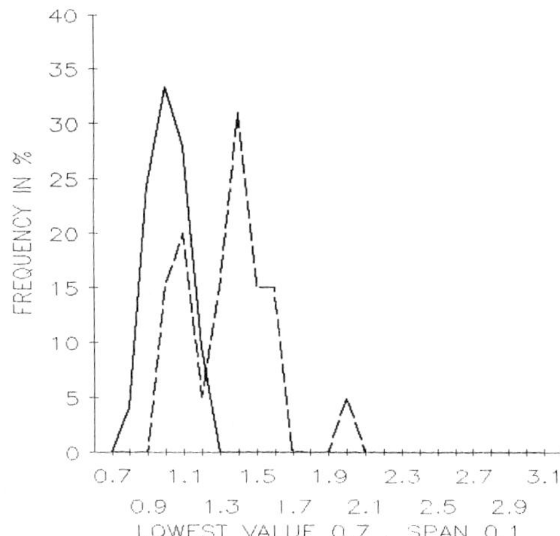

Fig. 1   **Fig. 2**

Fig. 1. Distribution of PR index values in 110 healthy patients (*solid line*), *85 common migraine patients (broken line)*, and 30 MCH patients (*dotted line*)

Fig. 2. Distribution of PR index values in 110 healthy patients (*solid line*) and 32 ergotamine headache patients (*broken line*)

Table 1. PR and subclassification of ergotamine headache

Clinical classification	(*n*)	PR index
Ergotamine headache	32	1.20±0.16
Types of headache after ergotamine withdrawal		
Migraine		
Common	18	1.36±0.16
Classical	–	–
Complicated	–	–
Muscle contraction headache	10	1.06±0.12
Unclassified	4	–

significantly different (*P* < 0.01) compared to PR of those suffering from common migraine (Table 1).

Discussion

The results indicate that common migraine is accompanied by alterations of platelet function. In contrast, PR in MCH was not different from headache-free controls. PR values in ergotamine headache were inconsistent. There is some evidence that platelets may play a role in migraine, but they cannot be exclusively responsible for the generation of headache.

The headache itself may be induced by a mediator, which can be influenced by ergotamine and a product of altered platelets as well. The common endpoint could be represented by the serotonin receptors in the vessel wall, which can be occupied by ergotamine (Saxena 1972; Müller-Schweinitzer 1978) and can be modulated by serotonin (Vanhoutte 1978; Edvinsson et al. 1983). In a similar way, release of platelet serotonin or decrease of ergotamine may affect the vessel wall serotonin receptors and induce the changes in cerebral blood flow (Simrad and Pausen 1973; Norris et al. 1975) observed during a migraine attack.

From the above results it is assumed that changes in platelet function observed during migraine-like ergotamine headaches depend on the underlying type of headache. There is evidence that ergotamine, even after long-term treatment, will not influence platelet reactivity – even if platelet aggregation seems to be changed by ergotamine (Hilton and Cumings 1972). In addition the results show that a migraine-like headache is possible without alteration of platelet reactivity.

Differences in PR between migraine plus ergotamine headache patients and MCH plus ergotamine headache patients are significant (Table 1). In clinical practice, however, these differences will not be useful as a diagnostic tool since the individual values overlap too much to allow a classification in each single case. From the clinical point of view it seems impressive that in an unselected group of 32 patients with ergotamine-induced headache, ten patients had never had a migraine headache and the original diagnosis in all patients referred was migraine headache.

References

Ad hoc committee on classification of headache (1962) Classification of headache. Arch Neurol 6:173–176

Born GVR (1982) Die Rolle der Thrombozyten bei der Athero- und Thrombogenese. Rheinisch Westfälische Akademie der Wissenschaften Nr 295 Sitzung Vortrag N320. Westdeutscher Verlag, Opladen

Deshmuk SV, Meyer JS (1977) Cyclic changes in platelet dynamics and the pathogenesis and prophylaxis of migraine. Postgrad Med 68,1:133–137

Edvinsson L, Degueurce A, Duverger D, MacKenzie ET, Scatton B, Uddman R (1983) Coupling between cerebral blood flow and metabolism: a role for serotonin? In: MacKenzie ET (ed) Neurotransmitters and the cerebral circulation 2:121–137

Grotemeyer KH, Hofferberth B (1985) Zirkulierende Plättchenaggregate bei Patienten mit akuten ischämischen und sogenannten chronischen zerebrovaskulären Störungen. Dtsch Med Wochenschr 110:256–259

Grotemeyer KH, Viand R, Beykirch K (1983) Thrombozytenfunktion bei vasomotorischem Kopfschmerz und Migränekopfschmerz. Dtsch Med Wochenschr 106:775–778

Hannington E, Jones R, Amess JAL, Wachowitz B (1981) Migraine a platelet disorder? Lancet II:720–721

Hilton BP, Cumings JN (1972) 5-Hydroxytryptamine levels and platelet aggregation responses in subjects with acute migraine headache. J Neurol Neurosurg Psychiatry 35:505–509

Kruglak L, Nathan I, Korczyn AD, Zolozov Z, Berginer V, Dvilansky A (1984) Platelet aggregability, disaggregability and serotonin uptake in migraine. Cephalalgia 4:221–225

Lechner H, Ott E, Fazekas E, Pilger E (1985) Evidence of enhanced platelet aggregation and platelet sensitivity in migraine patients. Cephalalgia 2:89–91

Müller-Schweinitzer E (1978) Studies on the 5-HT receptor in vascular smooth muscle. In: Friedman AP, Granger ME, Critchley M (eds) Research and clinical studies in headache, headache today – an update by 21 experts, vol 6:6–12. Karger, Basel
Norris JW, Hatchinski VC, Cooper PW (1975) Changes in cerebral blood flow during migraine attack. Br Med J [Clin Res] 3:676–677
Rose FC (1985) The role of platelets in migraine. Cephalalgia 2:83–85
Saxena PR (1972) The effects of antimigraine drugs on the vascular responses by 5-hydroxytryptamine and related biogenic substances on the external carotid bed of dogs: possible pharmacological implications to their antimigraine action. Headache 12:44–54
Simrad D, Paulsen OB (1973) Cerebral vasomotor paralysis during migraine attack. Arch Neurol 29:95–101
Vanhoutte PM (1978) Heterogenity in vascular smooth muscle. In: Kaley G, Altura BM (eds) Microcirculation. University press, Baltimore, pp 181–309

Treatment of Drug-Induced Headache

Short- and Long-Term Effects of Withdrawal Therapy in Drug-Induced Headache

H.-C. Diener, W. D. Gerber, S. Geiselhart, J. Dichgans, and E. Scholz

Introduction

Ergotamine preparations were used in the treatment of migraine attacks for the first time at the turn of this century. Between 1934 and 1946, Horton and co-workers performed several studies on the action of ergotamine, dihydroergotamine, and combinations with caffeine and barbiturates in the treatment of acute migraine attacks (Logan and Allen 1934; Horton et al. 1945, 1948; Peters 1953; Horton 1961). But already in 1951 (Peters and Horton 1951) and in a more extended study in 1963 (Horton and Peters 1963), the authors realized that patients with periodic headache (migraine and tension headache) who had used excessive amounts of ergotamine preparations for prolonged periods not only developed signs of ergotamine intoxication (vasospastic disturbances in the extremities, peripheral neuropathy), but in addition they also developed chronic headache.

The discontinuation of the drug resulted in withdrawal headache, a deterioration of the pre-existing chronic headache. After a time period of some days, headache was significantly improved (Horton and Peters 1963).

During the last 10 years, however, it has become evident that not only ergot preparations, but also many other analgesic drugs can lead to chronic headache (Lucas and Falkowski 1973; Tfelt-Hansen and Krabbe 1981; Isler 1982; Kudrow 1982; Wörz 1983; Dichgans et al. 1984; Rapaport et al. 1985; Henry et al. 1985). The combination of nonsteroidal anti-inflammatory drugs with ergotamine seems to be much more dangerous in this respect than the intake of single substances (Dichgans et al. 1984).

The aim of the present study was twofold: (a) with the use of headache diaries, we wanted to monitor in 1-h intervals the time course of headache and withdrawal symptoms after the abrupt discontinuance of drug intake; (b) in addition, we performed a long-term follow-up study in 85 patients with drug-induced headache after withdrawal therapy.

Department of Neurology, University of Tübingen, Liebermeisterstr. 18–20, D-7400 Tübingen, Federal Republic of Germany

Drug-Induced Headache
Ed. by H.-C. Diener and M. Wilkinson
© Springer-Verlag Berlin Heidelberg 1988

Results

Short-term Effects of Drug Withdrawal Therapy

This study included 27 patients with daily headache and chronic analgesic drug abuse. Women ($n=21$) outnumbered men ($n=6$) by a proportion of 3.5:1. All patients originally suffered from migraine. "Migraine" in this population was defined by recurrent attacks of headache, usually unilateral and associated with anorexia, nausea, and vomiting. In some patients attacks were preceded by or associated with neurological symptoms. The mean history of migraine was 14.7 years (range 3–40 years), the mean time interval of chronic daily headache was 5.9 years (range 1–26 years). The analysis of pain characteristics revealed diffuse and dull headache with the chracteristics of tension headache. Most patients reported a bilateral tight sensation in the head. This sensation was already present in the early morning. Most patients observed additional intermittent hemicrania with vegetative symptoms, reflecting migraine attacks superimposed on the analgesic headache.

All patients were informed about the symptoms of drug withdrawal prior to hospitalization. They were asked to keep headache diaries prior to and during withdrawal therapy. Headache intensity was scaled between 0 (no headache) and 5 (most intensive headache). Headache duration was measured in hours per day. In addition the patients reported subjective complaints. No analgesic, sedative, or prophylactic drugs were given during the first 10 days of withdrawal therapy.

The mean duration of headache was 18–19 h during the first 2 days, decreasing to 12 h on day 14 of withdrawal therapy (Fig. 1). The long duration of headache at the beginning of our recordings was due to rebound headache but could also be explained by sleep disturbances. Headache intensity increased sharply during the 1st day and then decreased more slowly from a mean value of 3.08 to

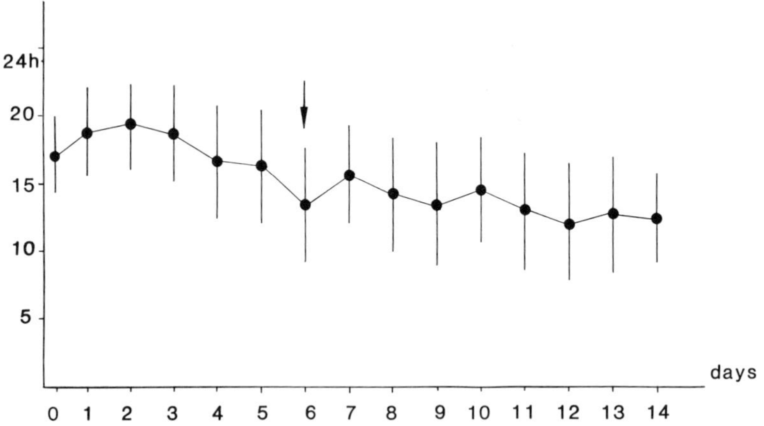

Fig. 1. Mean duration and standard deviations of headache within 24 h following abrupt stop of migraine and headache drug intake. The *arrow* indicates the significant decrease of headache duration from day 1 to day 6

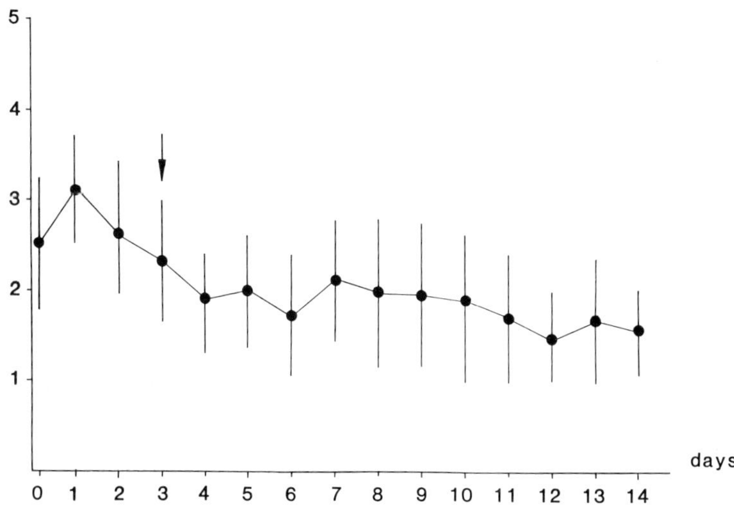

Fig. 2. Mean headache intensity on a scale from 0 (no headache) to 5 (most intensive headache) during drug withdrawal. Headache intensity was significantly improved on day 3 (*arrow*)

1.58 at day 14 (Fig. 2). Only very moderate withdrawal symptoms were experienced by 18% of the patients. The others experienced the typical rebound headache, which is localized in the neck and frontally with nausea, vomiting, sweating, tachycardia, vertigo, and insomnia. These side effects usually disappeared within 4–6 days. A total of 69% of the patients reported a very good or good improvement of headache at the end of the 2-week treatment period, 31% reported no change in the intensity and duration of headache.

Long-term Effects of Drug Withdrawal Therapy

This study included 85 patients with drug-induced headache. Preconditions to be included in the present study were: daily intake of analgesics or migraine drugs, more than 20 headache days per month, and a mean daily duration of headache of more than 12 h. The group under study consisted of 71 women and 14 men. The mean age was 44 years (range 21–70 years), the mean duration of drug-induced headache prior to withdrawal therapy was 6.1 years (range 0.5–38 years). The original headache was migraine in most cases (Table 1). All patients used drug combinations. Headache drugs in the Federal Republic of Germany are in most cases combinations of different analgesics like paracetamol, salicylic acid, and phenazone. Migraine drugs usually contain ergotamine, caffeine, barbiturates or codeine, and salicylic acid or acetaminophen. Substances most commonly used were caffeine, ergotamine, dihydroergotamine, barbiturates, and codeine. Most brands contained salicylic acid or acetaminophen.

All patients were hospitalized for 2 weeks and withdrawn from their analgesics or migraine drugs. Re-evaluation of migraine or tension headache was done in half of the cases by a personal standardized interview, in the remaining patients

Table 1. Clinical diagnosis of headache prior to analgesic abuse and mean duration of headache

Kind of headache	(n)	(%)	Mean (years)	Range (years)
Migraine	62	73	24.8	6–56
Migraine and tension headache	13	15	17.6	10–29
Tension headache	8	10	26.9	15–40
Post-traumatic headache	1	1	4	
Unknown	1	1	7	

by telephone interview. Patients were asked to scale headache parameters in relation to the month prior to withdrawal therapy. We recorded migraine attacks, tension headache, and drug-induced headache separately. Migraine attacks were defined as intermittent headache with vegetative or neurological disturbances. Tension headache was assumed when the patient reported a diffuse, dull headache with a tight sensation. Drug-induced headache was presumed when a daily headache was reported together with daily intake of analgesics. In addition, we asked for the intake of headache or migraine drugs during the last month.

The mean time interval of follow-up after therapy was 35 months (range 10–75 months). Success or failure of therapy was assessed by grouping patients into one of five different categories. Group A included patients who were totally free from headache and who did not use any headache medication. Group B was restricted to patients with intermittent migraine attacks, but with a significant reduction in the number of headache pills taken. If the number of headache days (either migraine or tension headache) was 50% or less compared to the prehospitalization time, and drug intake was reduced, the patient was included in group C. Patients in group D had no or only moderate improvement of headache.

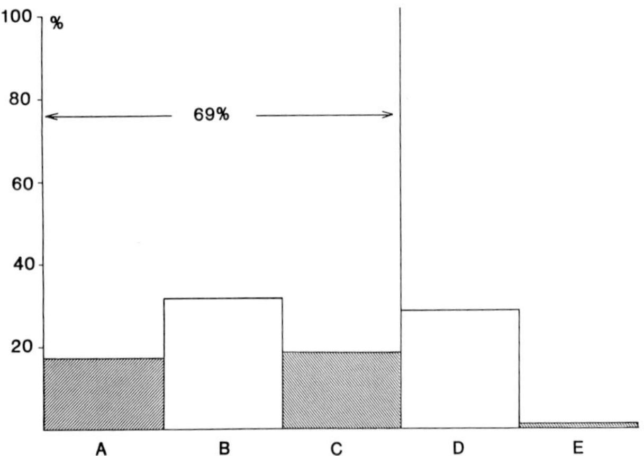

Fig. 3. Success or failure of drug withdrawal therapy after 2.9 years follow-up. Patients were assigned to groups A to E. *A*, no headache, no drugs; *B*, no daily headache, drugs <50%; *C*, headache 50% or less, drug intake 50% or less; *D*, headache >50%–100%; *E*, deterioration of headache. Groups A–C were considered to have gained from the therapy

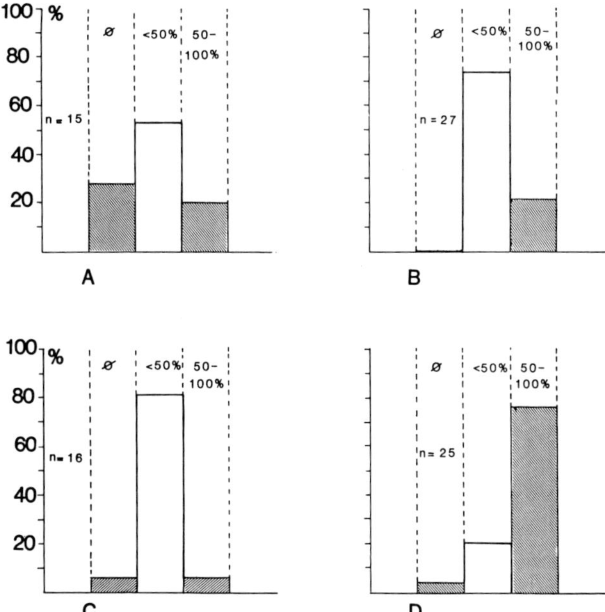

Fig. 4. Distribution of intensity and frequency of migraine attacks or tension headache attacks 2.9 years after drug withdrawal in groups A, B, C, and D (see Fig. 3). The *first column* shows patients without migraine or tension headache (0). The *middle column* shows how many patients scaled their headaches below 50% of original intensity or frequency (<50%). The *last column* indicates patients with insignificant or no improvement of original headache (50%–100%)

One patient (group E), who had relapsed, took more analgesics than prior to withdrawal therapy (Fig. 3). A total of 69% of the patients had a significant improvement of headache, 29.4% were unchanged, but only one patient had deteriorated. Drug withdrawal not only resulted in a relief of daily headache, but in addition, the frequency and intensity of the pre-existing migraine decreased. This improvement is shown in Fig. 4. Most patients had no difficulties in differentiating the characteristics of a typical migraine attack and drug-induced headache.

Closer Analysis

Barbiturates are known to result in dependency after prolonged use. We had therefore assumed that a bad outcome of withdrawal therapy could be related to the prior intake of barbiturates. A closer analysis of the drugs taken prior to withdrawal therapy and the success of this therapy showed no difference between the patients who had taken barbiturates and the ones who had not.

We asked the 26 patients who had an insignificant improvement of daily headache for possible reasons for the failure of our treatment. Most patients complained that we had sent them back to the referring physician after withdrawal without a concept of how to treat acute migraine attacks or how to perform migraine prophylaxis. This resulted in a change of our treatment strategy. Patients are now seen every 3 months by a neurologist and a psychologist, and treatment strategies including nonmedical treatment are developed. Six patients obviously had not understood the causal relationship between the intake of headache drugs and headache and were not really motivated to be withdrawn. Eight patients claimed that their headache was unchanged despite decreased intake of analgesics. Four patients reported that the intensity of their headache was not tolerable with the amount and kind of headache medication allowed by us. Five patients informed us that stress and fear of headache again resulted in prophylactic intake of migraine drugs. Three patients were not willing to give an explanation for their relapse.

Action of Prophylactic Treatment

All patients in this group had tried acupuncture treatment prior to withdrawal therapy. The positive effects of this therapy, if present, never lasted more than 3 months. Half the patients had prophylactic treatment with beta-blocking agents, calcium entry blockers, or serotonin antagonists prior to withdrawal. This prophylactic treatment was without any effect as long as these patients were still taking migraine drugs every day. In contrast, most of the patients still suffering from typical migraine attacks after withdrawal had significant therapeutic effects on migraine frequency and intensity when treated with metoprolol (50–200 mg/day) or flunarizine (5–10 mg/day). This result indicates that the daily intake of analgesics and migraine drugs counteracts the prophylactic action of beta-blocking drugs and calcium entry blockers.

Conclusions

Regular intake of analgesics and migraine drugs may lead to chronic headache with different characteristics from those of the original headache. All types of headache, e.g., migraine, tension, cluster, or post-traumatic headache can be the basis of regular drug intake. Tables 2–4 summarize the results reported in the literature about this specific form of headache. This kind of headache can be observed in many Western countries. Women are more frequently affected than men (Table 2). This reflects the fact that migraine occurs more frequently in women than in men (Bruyn 1985). An additional reason is the higher affinity of females to sedatives and tranquilizers with consequent drug dependency. Our own experience in 180 patients and a review of the literature indicate that all kinds of ergot derivates and analgesic/antipyretic combinations may cause chronic headache (Table 3). Drug combinations, especially those containing sedatives, hypnotics, and tranquilizers, are most dangerous, probably the latter ingredients promote dependency with inadvertent change in the goal of drug intake.

The success rate of withdrawal therapy in the literature is between 40% and 100%, with a mean rate of 70% depending on the time of follow-up, on the drugs

Table 2. Analgesic headache – review of the literature

Author	Year	Country	(n)	Women	Men
Ala-Hurula et al.	1982	SF	23	21	2
Andersson	1975	DK	44	39	5
Dichgans et al.	1984	FRG	52	48	4
Henry et al.	1985	F	22	17	5
Hokkanen et al.	1978	SF	43	37	6
Horton and Peters	1963	USA	52	22	30
Isler	1982	CH	104	71	33
Kudrow	1982	USA	200	167	33
Lucas and Falkowski	1973	GB	5	2	3
Rapaport et al.	1985	USA	90	69	21
Rowsell et al.	1973	GB	24	18	6
Tfelt-Hansen and Krabbe	1981	DK	40	35	5
Wörz	1983	FRG	80	46	34

taken, and on the original type of headache (Table 4). According to our experience, drug withdrawal is impossible on an outpatient basis in severe cases. Only three out of 200 patients were sucessful with the outpatient approach. Our patients are hospitalized in a neurological ward for a time period of 10–14 days. We discontinue drug intake abruptly and avoid all kinds of analgesics during the period of rebound headache in order to avoid a new conditioning and in order for the patient to experience the full range of drug-dependent rebound headache which is explained as one of the mechanisms of the previous daily headache. Headache is treated locally with ice cubes. On dismissal from the hospital, patients are instructed that they may use only salicylic acid or acetaminophen in combination with metoclopramide for the treatment of acute migraine attacks. Ergotamine is restricted to patients who, despite this regimen, still suffer from severe migraine attacks. Cumulative ergotamine intake (only monosubstances) is restricted to 4 mg during one attack and to 14 mg during a month. Drugs containing caffeine, phenazone, barbiturates, antihistamines, and codeine are strictly forbidden as well as all kinds of drug combinations.

The decision about prophylactic drug and/or behavioral treatment is made 3 months after withdrawal on the basis of headache diaries. Patients with more than two migraine attacks within 1 month or attacks lasting longer than 36 h are first treated with metoprolol (initially 50 mg/day, then 100–200 mg/day). In patients in whom this treatment is unsuccessful after 3 months, we use either propranolol (80–200 mg/day) or flunarizine (5–10 mg/day). In this patient group, we never use dihydrated ergot preparations for migraine prophylaxis.

Summary

Regular intake of analgesics and migraine drugs may result in daily headache. The only successful therapy is drug withdrawal on an inpatient basis. A review of the literature shows success rates in terms of relief of headache in about 70%

Table 3. Analgesic headache – patients taking a single substance

Author	Ergot-amine (%)	Dihydro-ergotamine (%)	Caf-feine (%)	Barbi-turates (%)	Code-ine (%)	ASS (%)	Phen-acetin (%)	Acet-aminophen (%)	Others (%)
Ala-Hurula et al.	100		100	44					100
Andersson	100								
Dichgans et al.	52	28	96	73	50	48	55	48	50
Henry et al.	27		77	54		13		9	81
Hokkanen et al.	100								
Horton and Peters	100	2	66	26			6		26
Isler	——— 78 ———						21		
Kudrow				66	97		28		19
Lucas and Falkowski	100		20	20					18
Rapaport et al.						100	100		
Rowsell et al.	100								
Tfelt-Hansen and Krabbe	100		100	100					100
Wörz	35	25	71	100	40	30	53		28

Table 4. Analgesic headache – results of drug withdrawal therapy

Author	Year	Follow-up (months)	Positive results (%)
Ala-Hurula et al.	1982	3–6	78
Andersson	1975	6	82
Dichgans et al.	1984	16	77
Henry et al.	1985	3	78
Hokkanen et al.	1978	?	?
Horton and Peters	1963	?	100
Isler	1982	1–30	78
Kudrow	1982	1	60
Lucas and Falkowski	1973	1	40
Rapaport et al.	1985	3	67
Rowsell et al.	1973	1	100
Tfelt-Hansen and Krabbe	1981	12	72
Wörz	1983	?	?

of the patients within a follow-up period between 1 and 30 months. In the present study, we monitored headache intensity and duration during withdrawal therapy in 27 patients. The abrupt stop of analgesic intake resulted in a significant decrease of headache intensity at day 3 and of daily headache duration at day 6 of therapy.

The long-term effects of drug withdrawal therapy were evaluated in a population of 85 patients (71 women, 14 men). The precondition to be included in this study was to suffer from headache for more than 20 days a month. A total of 73% of these patients originally suffered from migraine, the others from migraine in combination with tension headache, tension headache only, or post-traumatic headache. The mean duration of the original headache (e.g., migraine) was 24.8 years, the duration of daily headache 6.1 years. The average daily intake of headache or migraine drugs in one single patient was 2.8. All patients took drug combinations. A total of 69% of the patients improved significantly (headache 50% or less, drug intake 50% or less compared to pretreatment) 35 months (range 10–75 months) after withdrawal therapy. A total of 18% of the patients were free from headache.

References

Ala-Hurula V, Myllylä V, Hokkanen E (1982) Ergotamine abuse: results of ergotamine discontinuation with special reference to the plasma concentrations. Cephalalgia 2:189–195

Andersson PG (1975) Ergotamine headache. Headache 15:118–121

Bruyn GW (1985) Prevalence and incidence of migraine – a critical review. In: Carroll JD, Pfaffenrath V, Sjaastad O (eds) Migraine and beta-blockers. Hässle, Mölndal, pp 99–109

Dichgans J, Diener HC, Gerber WD, Verspohl EJ, Kukiolka H, Kluck M (1984) Analgetika-induzierter Dauerkopfschmerz. Dtsch Med Wochenschr 109:369–373

Henry P, Dartigues JF, Benetier MP, Lucas J, Duplan B, Jogeix M, Orgogozo JM (1985) Ergotamine- and analgesic-induced headaches. In: Rose FC (ed) Migraine. Proceedings 5th International Migraine Symposion London 1984. Karger, Basel, pp 197–205

Hokkanen E, Waltimo O, Kallaurata T (1978) Toxic effects of ergotamine used for migraine. Headache 18:95–98

Horton BT (1961) Histaminic cephalgia (Horton's headache or syndrome). Md State Med J 10:178–203

Horton BT, Peters GA (1963) Clinical manifestations of excessive use of ergotamine preparations and management of withdrawal effect: report of 52 cases. Headache 3:214–226

Horton BT, Peters GA, Blumenthal LS (1945) A new product in the treatment of migraine: a preliminary report. Proc Staff Meet Mayo Clin 20:241–248

Horton BT, Ryan R, Reynolds JL (1948) Clinical observations on the use of E.C.110, a new agent for the treatment of headache. Proc Staff Meet Mayo Clin 23:105–108

Isler H (1982) Migraine treatment as a cause of chronic migraine. In: Rose FC (ed) Advances in migraine research and therapy. Raven, New York, pp 159–164

Kudrow L (1982) Paradoxical effects of frequent analgesic use. In: Critchley M, Friedman AP, Gorini S, Sicuteri F (eds) Advances in neurology, vol 33. Raven, New York, pp 335–341

Logan AH, Allen EV (1934) The treatment of migraine with ergotamine tartrate. Proc Staff Meet Mayo Clin 9:585–588

Lucas RN, Falkowski W (1973) Ergotamine and methysergide abuse in patients with migraine. Br J Psychiatry 122:199–203

Peters GA (1953) Migraine. Diagnosis and treatment with emphasis on the migraine-tension headache, provocative tests and use of rectal suppositories. Proc Staff Meet Mayo Clin 28:673–686

Peters GA, Horton BT (1951) Headache: with special reference to the excessive use of ergotamine preparations and withdrawal effects. Proc Staff Meet Mayo Clin 26:153–161

Rapaport A, Weeks R, Schaftell F (1985) Analgesic rebound headache: theoretical and practical implications. In: Olesen J, Tfelt-Hansen P, Jensen K (eds) Headache 85. Proceedings Second International Headache Congress. Jensen, Copenhagen, pp 448–449

Rowsell AR, Neylan C, Wilkinson M (1973) Ergotamine induced headache in migrainous patients. Headache 13:65–67

Tfelt-Hansen P, Krabbe AE (1981) Ergotamine abuse. Do patients benefit from withdrawal? Cephalagia 1:29–32

Wörz R (1983) Effects and risks of psychotropic and analgesic combinations. Am J Med 11:139–140

Wörz R, Baar H, Draf W, Garcia J, Gerbershagen HU, Gross D, Margin F, Ritter K, Scheifele J, Scholl W (1975) Kopfschmerz in Abhängigkeit von Analgetika-Mischpräparaten. Münch Med Wochenschr 177:457–462

Therapeutic Approach to Drug Abuse in Headache Patients

G. C. Manzoni [1], G. Micieli [2], F. Granella [1], G. Sandrini [2],
C. Zanferrari [1], and G. Nappi [2]

Introduction

The therapeutic approach to headache patients who abuse medications, in particular analgesics, represents a special challenge for the clinician. Hospitalization in a headache unit is, in fact, frequently required because it provides the opportunity to discontinue the analgesics abused and to attend to the sometimes severe consequences of abuse (Saper 1983). On the other hand, an exact definition of the clinical form of headache, in each case presenting with a more or less chronic pattern, is also required in order to develop an appropriate prophylactic treatment. The pharmacological approach will be based, in turn, on drugs with antimigraine properties to treat the so-called migraine with interparoxysmal headache (MIH), while anxyolitic and/or antidepressive compounds will be used to prevent the onset of chronic tension headache (CTH). These two clinical entities, as described elsewhere in this volume (Micieli et al.), are also characterized by aspects of drug abuse sometimes completely different from each other so that discontinuance of the drugs abused may need different procedures.

In the last few years, some models of therapeutic approach to analgesic and/or ergotamine abuse have been proposed (Lippmann 1955; Andersson 1975; Tfelt-Hansen and Krabbe 1981; Ala-Hurula et al. 1981, 1982; Kudrow 1982; Barolin 1983; Henry et al. 1984). However, the limited number of patients treated and the absence of diagnostic criteria which really fit the clinical features of the different forms of daily chronic headache have probably prevented, at least in some cases, adequate clinical responses. In particular, in a previous trial conducted by our group the nonsteroidal anti-inflammatory drug ketoprofen was used on a patient population suffering from daily chronic headache, and its efficacy was assessed in comparison with diazepam, a benzodiazepine frequently prescribed in these cases because of its myorelaxant and anxyolitic properties (Micieli et al. 1982). The experimental design consisted of two alternating periods in the same patient separated by 7 wash-out days. Ketoprofen was able to reduce pain parameters (duration and severity) and to maintain a constant effect of statistical significance, in comparison to pretreatment values, during the observation period.

The effects of diazepam seemed less marked and significant, being in any case independent of the wake-sleep phases. An important finding was also represented by the outcome of the analgesic consumption index which showed no significant

[1] Headache Center, Department of Neurology, University of Parma, Via del Quartiere 4, 43100 Parma, Italy
[2] Headache Center, Department of Neurology, C. Mondino Foundation, University of Pavia, Via Palestro 3, 27100 Pavia, Italy

Drug-Induced Headache
Ed. by H.-C. Diener and M. Wilkinson
© Springer-Verlag Berlin Heidelberg 1988

changes, probably indicating that the pain tolerance remained unchanged even in the presence of an actual reduction of pain severity and duration, suggesting at the same time a "peripheral" mechanism of action of both drugs used.

In that study no diagnostic attempt was made to detect either migrainous or muscle contraction forms of daily chronic headache. A similar distinction was made in another study in which the Ca^{2+} entry blocker flunarizine and the prostaglandin synthetase inhibitor indoprofen were administered to MIH and CTH patients with elevated headache scores in order to define the pharmacological and/or biochemical profile of responsive patients (Micieli et al. 1985).

In this study, flunarizine was able to reduce the pain total index (PTI) (sum of daily number of headache hours quantified on the basis of pain intensity: score 0–3), attack frequency, and analgesic consumption, and to increase the number of headache-free days in over 85% of the cases by the end of a 6-month open trial in which this drug was administered in single doses of 10 mg/day at bedtime.

On the other hand, in a controlled double-blind cross-over trial versus placebo during two 30-day treatment periods separated by a wash-out phase of 7 days, a significant response to indoprofen was observed in a smaller number of patients (30.7% of the cases). In the CTH group no difference was found between placebo and indoprofen treatments, while in MIH a reduction of PTI, which continued through the following phase, could be found when indoprofen preceded placebo.

The different responses of MIH and CTH to indoprofen are difficult to explain even if subsequent neurobiological and neurophysiological investigations seem to point to a different involvement of the pain control system in these two headache pathologies, characterized by a more severe impairment in MIH patients (Nappi et al. 1985; Sandrini et al. 1986). The results of these trials also confirm indirectly the data demonstrating different characteristics of analgesic abuse in MIH and CTH patients (Micieli et al. this volume). In the same way, MIH and CTH abusers could be supposed to exhibit a different pattern in the analgesic withdrawal syndrome, at least when considering the different characteristics of duration and quality of chronic drug intake.

Subjects and Methods

In this study 21 consecutive headache patients who were found to be drug abusers (i.e., having taken analgesics every day for at least 1 year) were hospitalized for detoxification and submitted to a support therapy during the so-called withdrawal syndrome. The distribution by sex and type of headache of the patients admitted to the study is shown in Table 1. According to the criteria described before (Micieli et al. this volume), 17 subjects (12 females and five males) suffered from MIH, while four had CTH. Moreover, both headache groups showed a clear female prevalence. Table 2 gives details of the course of headache in these patients.

No difference is observed between MIH and CTH subjects when age at first observation, age at headache onset, and duration of the episodic pattern of head-

Table 1. Population studied. Distribution by sex and type of headache

	Females ($n=15$)		Males ($n=6$)		Total ($n=21$)	
	(n)	(%)	(n)	(%)	(n)	(%)
MIH	12	70.5	5	29.5	17	100.0
CTH	3	75.0	1	25.0	4	100.0

Table 2. Population studied. Course of headache

	MIH ($n=17$)		CTH ($n=4$)		Total ($n=21$)
	Mean	Range	Mean	Range	Mean
Age at first observation (years)	45.4	26–61	52.7	35–68	47.3
Age at headache onset (years)	19.3	5–50	21.6	9–45	19.9
Duration of episodic headache (years)	22.0	1–46	22.3	7–35	22.1
Duration of chronic phase (years)	4.2	1–18	8.8	1–23	5.1

ache are considered. On the other hand, the two groups of patients seem to have a different duration of the chronic phase which is longer in CTH. Only a limited number of patients abused drugs containing ergotamine. In fact, among the 21 patients studied, five (23.8%) were abusers of this type of drug, while an equal number of the others consumed ergotamine-free analgesics with barbiturates (eight cases) and without barbiturates (eight cases). Moreover, MIH patients were more frequently heavy abusers either of ergotamine-free drugs or of ergotamine compounds, as seen when computing the weekly amount of analgesics in each group (Table 3).

When the drugs abused were withdrawn, a standardized support therapy was started from the 1st day of withdrawal (Fig. 1). This treatment included fluid replacement substances, analgesics (indomethacin, 50 mg twice a day i.v.), antiemetics (metoclopramide, 10 mg i.m., if required), tranquilizers (bromazepam 3 mg p.o. twice a day) and sleep inducers (triazolam 0.5 mg p.o. at bedtime). These drugs were usually administered for about 10 days in all cases.

Table 3. Weekly amounts of instant relief drugs taken by patients ($n=21$)

	Ergotamine-free analgesics (dose/week)			Ergotamine-containing drugs (mg/week)		
	10	10–20	20	10	10–24	24
MIH	1	3	8	–	3	2
CTH	2	1	1			
Total	3	4	9			

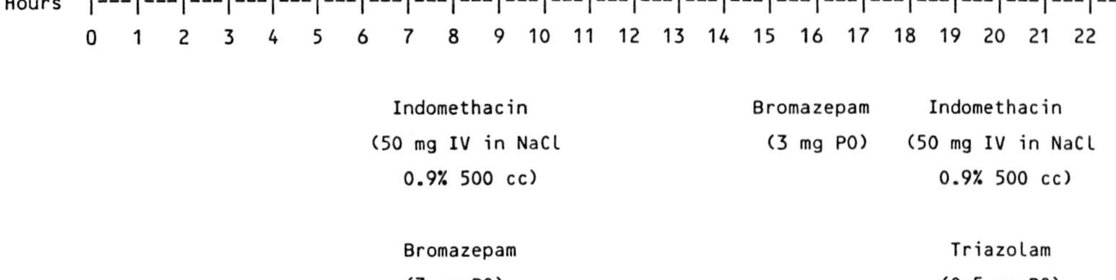

Fig. 1. Support therapy (standard schedule)

At the end of the detoxification period, almost all the subjects had prophylactic treatment. The choice was limited in these cases to flunarizine (at a daily dosage of 10 mg at bedtime) or amitriptyline (at the dosage of 75 mg t.i.d.). The follow-up time was 6 months for all the patients.

The distribution by headache form of the different treatments adopted is reported in Table 4. The abrupt discontinuation of the drugs abused induced withdrawal symptoms within 48 h in all the patients we studied. The clinical features of this withdrawal syndrome were similar to those reported in the literature for ergotamine discontinuation (Andersson 1975; Ala-Hurula et al. 1981; Diener et al. 1983). Furthermore, the symptoms our patients complained of were the same in all of them, regardless of the drug used. In particular, a severe headache ("rebound" headache) described as the most painful ever experienced, was reported in 88% of MIH cases, but it was also observed in two subjects suffering from CTH. Nausea, anxiety, and insomnia were also reported with the same frequency by the patients in both headache groups. However, only MIH abusers showed, in some cases, a slight increase in blood pressure and a moderate rise in body temperature for 2–4 days after drug discontinuation (Table 9).

The withdrawal symptoms lasted from 3 to 7 days. It was obvious that some of the differences observed between the two headache groups regarding the clinical characteristics of the discontinuation could be ascribed to the type of drug abused. In fact, the patients who abused ergotamine always showed a severe rebound headache, together with a higher incidence of other features (hypertension, hyperthermia) during the withdrawal period. On the other hand, a severe head-

Table 4. Prophylactic treatment

	MIH ($n=17$)	CTH ($n=4$)
Flunarizine (10 mg daily for 3 months)	10	–
Amitriptyline (75 mg daily for 3 months)	4	3
No treatment	3	1

Table 5. Withdrawal syndrome in MIH and CTH patients

MIH ($n=17$)	(n)	(%)	CTH ($n=4$) (n)	(%)	Total ($n=21$) (n)	(%)
Rebound headache (mild or moderate)	2	11.8	2	50.0	4	19.1
Rebound headache (severe or very severe)	15	88.2	2	50.0	17	80.9
Nausea	14	82.3	3	75.0	17	80.9
Vomiting	11	64.7	1	25.0	12	57.1
Anxiety	9	52.9	2	50.0	11	52.3
Insomnia	12	70.5	3	75.0	15	71.4
Blood pressure increase	4	23.5	–	–	4	19.1
Fever	2	11.7	–	–	2	9.5

Table 6. Withdrawal syndrome in ergot and nonergot abusers

	Ergotamine-containing drugs ($n=5$) (n)	(%)	Ergotamine-free with barbiturates ($n=8$) (n)	(%)	Analgesics: without barbiturates ($n=8$) (n)	(%)
Rebound headache (mild or moderate)	–	–	1	12.5	3	37.5
Rebound headache (severe or very severe)	5	100.0	7	87.5	5	62.5
Nausea	5	100.0	7	87.5	5	62.5
Vomiting	5	100.0	4	50.0	3	37.5
Anxiety	5	100.0	4	50.0	2	25.0
Insomnia	4	80.0	6	75.0	5	62.5
Blood pressure increase	4	80.0	–	–	–	–
Fever	2	40.0	–	–	–	–

ache also characterized the discontinuance of nonergotamine compounds containing barbiturates, while it was less frequently reported by the patients taking barbiturate-free analgesics (Table 6).

The results of this "acute" treatment of analgesic abuse were excellent and characterized by a marked reduction in frequency and severity indices of headache symptomatology. At the end of this 10-day therapy, in fact, all the patients were completely free of headache or reported dramatic reduction. Three subjects suffering from MIH before discontinuation of analgesics as well as a patient exhibiting a pure "tension" form of daily chronic headache did not receive any longtime treatment because they showed almost complete pain relief, characterized by marked reduction in the frequency of migraine attacks (less than 1 per month) or by the absence of tension headache episodes.

The 6-month follow-up was characterized by low relapse rate (22.2%). Good results were observed, in particular, among MIH patients, who showed a percentage improvement of monthly PTI between 40% and 60% in five cases and over 60% in the remaining cases, whereas, among CTH patients, two of four subjects did not show any significant improvements during these treatments. It is worth noting that none of our patients received any benefit from the prophylactic treatments (mostly with Ca^{2+} entry blockers, beta-blockers or pizotifen) started in the year before the detoxification period, thus suggesting that no drugs seem to be effective while analgesics are still being abused.

Conclusion

The need for a distinction among the chronic forms of headache, at least those with "migrainous," "tension," or (also for the obvious absence of drug abuse) psychogenic characteristics, is the first point emerging from our data. As reported (Micieli et al. this volume), patients with MIH exhibit clinical features and characteristics of abuse which are sometimes very different from those of the subjects suffering from CTH, even if some of these features, such as the female preponderance among MIH patients, may be considered as part of the clinical picture of migraine syndromes. In the same way these two groups of headache patients are likely to show different withdrawal symptomatology and long-term response to prophylactic treatment. In any case, however, the abrupt discontinuation of the drugs abused seems to represent the most advisable decisions to make for the treatment of physical and/or psychological dependence on analgesics.

The clinical features of the withdrawal syndrome suggest that hospitalization is required in many cases for the treatment of "rebound" headache, as well as for the most appropriate psychological approach to the problem of analgesic abuse/dependence. Moreover, analgesic abuse is often related to the deficiency of pain control mechanisms as demonstrated, at least among MIH patients, by decreased endorphinergic activity (Genazzani et al. 1984; Nappi et al. 1985) and impairment of nociceptive threshold and tolerance (Sandrini et al. 1986), which show a direct correlation with the severity of headache. On the other hand, this type of drug abuse resembles in some cases a "compulsive" habit, suggesting analogies with disorders of seeking behavior. Traumatic life events, depressive episodes, or "neuroticism" could also favor the onset of analgesic abuse, at least in some headache subgroups. Thus, further studies are necessary to define more accurately the profile of chronic headache patients. Among these, the major interest lies in the subjects suffering from a "pure" muscle contraction form of CTH, in whom the earliest onset of a chronic pattern, the abuse of drugs other than analgesics, and the poor response to prophylactic treatment seem to characterize peculiar and really differentiated psychobiological and pharmacological profiles.

Summary

Twenty-one consecutive headache patients, who were found to be drug abusers, were hospitalized for detoxification and subjected to a support therapy during the so-called withdrawal syndrome. This syndrome, frequently characterized by severe headache, nausea, vomiting, anxiety, and insomnia, lasted a total of 3–7 days. Analgesics, antiemetics, and tranquilizers were administered for 10 days as support therapy along with fluid replacement substances. The results were excellent, and at the end of treatment all patients were completely free of headache or had it dramatically reduced. The 6-month follow-up showed a low rclapse rate (22.2%). Drug abuse had been among the potential factors favoring a transformation of the headache in all patients who were still symptom-free 6 months after withdrawal.

References

Ala-Hurula U, Myllylä VV, Hokkanen E, Tokda O (1981) Tolfenamic acid and ergotamine abuse. Headache 21:240–242

Ala-Hurula U, Myllylä VV, Hokkanen E (1982) Ergotamine abuse: results of ergotamine discontinuation, with special reference to the plasma concentration. Cephalalgia 2:189–195

Andersson P (1975) Ergotamine headache. Headache 15:118–121

Barolin GS (1983) Chronified headache and its treatment. 1st Int Headache Congress, 14–16 Sept 1983, Munich (Abstr book, p 131)

Diener HC, Dichgans J, Gerber WD, Kuriolka H (1983) Drug induced chronic headache. 1st Int Headache Congress, 14–16 Sept 1983, Munich (Abstr book, p 130)

Genazzani AR, Nappi G, Facchinetti F, Micieli G, Petraglia F, Bono G, Monittola C, Savoldi F (1984) Progressive impairment of CSF B-EP levels in migraine sufferers. Pain 18:127–133

Henry P, Dartigues JF, Benetier MP, Lucas J, Duplan B, Jogeix M, Orgogozo JM (1984) Ergotamine- and analgesic-induced headaches. Controlled study of the use of electrical stimulation of high frequency current. In: Rose FC (ed) Migraine. Karger, Basel, pp 197–205

Kudrow L (1982) Paradoxical effect of frequent analgesic use. In: Critchley M, Friedman AP, Gorini S, Sicuteri F (eds) Advances in neurology, vol 33. Raven, New York, pp 335–341

Lippmann CW (1955) Characteristic headache resulting from prolonged use of ergot derivatives. J Nerv Ment Dis 121:270–273

Micieli G, Sances G, Cerutti G, Sinforiani E, Bono G (1982) Therapeutic approach to chronic daily headache patients. Int J Clin Pharm Res 2:135–142

Micieli G, Piazza D, Sinforiani E, Cavallini A, Trucco M, Gabellini S, Mancuso A, Pacchetti C (1985) Antimigraine drugs in the management of daily chronic headaches: clinical profiles of responsive patients. Cephalalgia 5 [Suppl 2]:219–224

Nappi G, Facchinetti F, Martignoni E, Petraglia F, Manzoni GC, Sances G, Sandrini G, Genazzani AR (1985) Endorphin patterns within the headache spectrum disorders. Cephalalgia 5 [Suppl 2]:201–210

Sandrini G, Martignoni E, Micieli G, Alfonsi E, Sances G, Nappi G (1986) Pain reflexes in the clinical assessment of migraine syndromes. Funct Neurol 1/4:423–429

Saper JR (1983) Headache disorder. Current concepts and treatment strategies. Wright, Boston

Tfelt-Hansen P, Krabbe AA (1981) Ergotamine abuse. Do patients benefit from withdrawal? Cephalalgia 1:29–32

Management of Ergotamine Withdrawal

N. T. Mathew

Excessively frequent use of ergotamine is known to produce a number of complications which interfere with the effective management of patients with chronic recurrent headaches. It is known to produce malaise, nausea and, above all, increased frequency of headache (Lippman 1955; Saper 1967; Rose and Wilkinson 1976), and subsequently a predictable daily or near daily headache syndrome (Mathew et al. 1982). The therapeutic range becomes progressively narrower with long-term usage of ergotamine. Chronic abuse of ergotamine also produces ergotism which has a number of manifestations including involvement of the cardiovascular system, apparently secondary to arterial spasm in the major arterial territories, especially in the limbs; and neurological manifestations such as confusion, psychosis, convulsions, drowsiness, hemiplegia and peripheral neuropathy (Hokkanen et al. 1978; Horton and Peters 1982).

Severe withdrawal symptoms are often reported on discontinuation of ergotamine (Friedman et al. 1955; Lippman 1955; Rowsell et al. 1973). The symptoms include increased headache, nausea, vomiting, excitement, sleeplessness, and even hallucinations. From the previous studies it appears that there are individual variations in the development of toxic and withdrawal symptoms. Those who take more than 10 mg of ergotamine in a week are at increased risk of developing either of these groups of problems. It is a common clinical observation that patients who are on an excessively chronic use of ergotamine do not respond to other prophylactic antimigraine agents unless ergotamine is withdrawn first.

Strategies in Ergotamine Withdrawal

Development of toxic symptoms and ergotamine rebound headaches are both indications for withdrawal of ergotamine. The techniques of withdrawal vary from center to center. In general, it can be accomplished in an outpatient or an inpatient setting. Ergotamine can be withdrawn abruptly or gradually. It should be pointed out that chronic headache patients who are on ergotamine may also be on other analgesic/caffeine/sedative/narcotic combinations for the relief of pain, and some of these medications are known to cause rebound phenomena and increased headache (Kudrow 1982). Therefore, a complete drug withdrawal program may be in order for these patients.

Houston Headache Clinic, 1213 Hermann Dr. Suite 350, Houston, TX 77004, USA

Drug-Induced Headache
Ed. by H.-C. Diener and M. Wilkinson
© Springer-Verlag Berlin Heidelberg 1988

Outpatient Versus Inpatient Withdrawal Programs

Some centers accomplish the withdrawal of ergotamine in an outpatient setting as a gradual process over a period of weeks. Disadvantages of outpatient programs are poor compliance and long withdrawal periods. The main advantage of the outpatient program is the lower cost. Since sudden withdrawal of ergotamine may cause a number of unpleasant symptoms, such an approach may not be suitable for outpatient programs in all cases. Any program, whether outpatient or inpatient, should be combined with behavioral therapy which will help patients in the total management of their headache syndrome.

We prefer inpatient withdrawal programs for withdrawal of ergotamine and other symptomatic medications in chronic headache patients because (a) it insures compliance; (b) the severe withdrawal symptoms can be counteracted easily in an inpatient setting; (c) withdrawal can be accomplished fairly rapidly; (d) while the withdrawal is accomplished, prophylactic medications can be initiated and dosages adjusted; and (e) an intensive behavioral approach can be instituted during the inpatient withdrawal period.

Amelioration of Ergotamine Withdrawal Symptoms

Various therapies have been used in the management of ergotamine withdrawal symptoms. Hydration with intravenous fluid therapy and antinausea medications are essential if the withdrawal is done rapidly. The usual practice is to employ narcotic analgesics and sedatives to counteract the withdrawal symptoms. One should be extremely careful in using habit-forming medications as there is a distinct danger of substituting one habituation for another. In the past, various other therapies have been recommended for the weaning period. Andersson et al. (1975) used antiserotonin agents and light sedatives. Lippman (1955) found that corticosteroids were useful in the amelioration of symptoms of ergotamine withdrawal. Tfelt-Hansen and Krabbe (1981) used levopromazine for the management of ergotamine abuse. Based on the previous reports of the use of Limoge current in aiding withdrawal of narcotics from drug addicts, Henry et al. (1984) studied its effects on patients undergoing ergotamine withdrawal. They found no beneficial effect from Limoge current in their patients.

Ala-Hurula et al. (1981) reported the effectiveness of tolfenamic acid, a nonsteroidal anti-inflammatory agent, in preventing the recurrence of ergotamine abuse. Tolfenamic acid has also been used effectively in the treatment of acute migraine. Naproxen has recently been studied in the prophylaxis of migraine (Welch et al. 1985) and is a useful adjunct in the management of chronic mixed headache syndrome. A study of the effectiveness of naproxen in the management of ergotamine withdrawal was undertaken at the Houston Headache Clinic.

Patients

A total of 22 patients hospitalized for ergotamine withdrawal were randomly allocated to two groups. Group A consisted of ten patients in whom ergotamine was withdrawn with the use of only symptomatic medication such as antiemetics, analgesics, and hydration. Group B consisted of 12 patients who were started on naproxen, 500 mg, 1 day before the withdrawal was initiated and continued until the withdrawal was complete.

Observations were made starting 4 days before the withdrawal was initiated and was continued for 8 days afterwards. The patients were hospitalized on the day of withdrawal. Prior to admission to the hospital, patients were given a headache diary in which they noted the intensity of the headache on a 1–10 scale, the duration of headache at different intensities, the associated symptoms such as nausea, vomiting, and amount of antiemetics and analgesics they used during that period. They were asked to assess their total sleep time and note down any sedatives, tranquilizers, or hypnotics they used during that period.

After admission to the hospital, a similar diary was maintained by the patients in addition to the physicians' and nurses' records on the above parameters. Careful documentation was made on the amount of analgesics, antiemetics, sedatives, and tranquilizers used during the withdrawal period. Three patients could not tolerate naproxen beyond 2 days and were therefore excluded from the study.

Results

The age, sex, duration of headache, diagnostic category, and toxic effects of ergotamine are shown in Tables 1 and 2. Figure 1 shows the effect of concomitant use of naproxen on the headache index in both groups. Headache index was calculated by multiplying the severity of headache on a 1–10 scale by the duration of headache for each severity for a 24-h period. It should be noted that the maximum increase of headache was on the 2nd, 3rd, and 4th days after withdrawal. Group B on naproxen had significantly fewer headaches than Group A ($P < 0.01$).

Figure 2 shows the number of analgesic tablets consumed by the patient during the observation period. These include a total of all the analgesic medications taken by the patient as it was not possible to categorize them because there was no uniformity in the type of medication they took. It is evident from Fig. 2 that the use of analgesic medications increased in Group A on the 2nd, 3rd, and 4th days of withdrawal. Group B used a significantly smaller number of analgesic tablets.

Figure 3 shows the amount of antiemetics (promethazine) used by the patient. There was an increase in use of promethazine on the 2nd, 3rd, and 4th days corresponding to the increased headache. The concomitant use of naproxen reduced the need for larger doses of antiemetics.

An indirect measure of restlessness, total sleep time, was evaluated (Fig. 4). Group B had significantly more total sleep time during the withdrawal period

Table 1. Ergotamine overuse (Group A – control)

Age	Sex	Diagnosis	Duration of headache (years)	Average weekly dose of ergotamine (mg)	Toxic symptoms
55	F	Common migraine	18	10	Daily headache confusion
40	F	Common migraine	4	16	Chest pain, paresthesia, muscle pain, daily headache, depression
29	M	Classic migraine	6	12	Increased headache frequency
38	F	Mixed headache	12	8	Paresthesia
28	M	Mixed headache	4	14	Depression, chest pain, arterial spasms, lower extensor muscle ache
50	F	Common migraine	18	10	Daily headache
42	F	Common migraine	5	14	Poor memory, confusion Parethesia
61	F	Mixed headache	30	12	Intermittent claudication
64	F	Common migraine	14	15	Sleeplessness, poor memory, confusion, parethesia, muscle pain
32	F	Common migraine	3	19	Increased headache
Mean 44			11	12	

Table 2. Ergotamine overuse (Group B – naproxen)

Age	Sex	Diagnosis	Duration of headache (years)	Average weekly dose of ergotamine (mg)	Toxic symptoms
44	F	Common migraine	21	14	Paresthesia, daily Headache
45	M	Cluster Headache	12	28	Ischemic symptoms, spasms of both brachial arteries
51	F	Common migraine	14	12	Daily headache
63	F	Common migraine	27	14	Chest pain, confusion
61	F	Common migraine	24	10	Sleeplessness, confusion, malaise
55	F	Mixed headache	30	10	Gastric symptoms
34	F	Common migraine	4	12	Muscle aches, daily headache
58	M	Mixed headache	16	16	Paresthesia, pigmented skin lesion
48	F	Common headache	22	12	Daily headache
38	F	Mixed headache	6	14	Cold ext. sweating chest pain
49	F	Common migraine	12	10	Gastric symptoms, nausea daily headache
32	M	Classic migraine	5	16	Increased headaches
Mean 48			16	14	

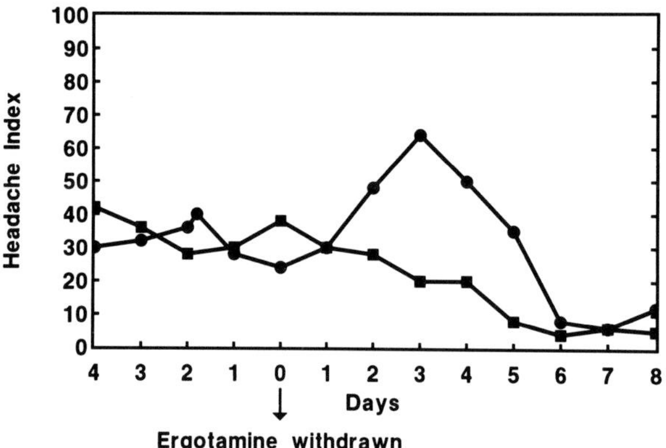

Fig. 1. Ergotamine withdrawal, effect of concomitant use of naproxen on the daily headache index (severity × duration). Note the maximum increased headache between 2nd and 5th days after withdrawal of ergotamine. *Circles*, control ($n=10$); *squares*, naproxen ($n=12$)

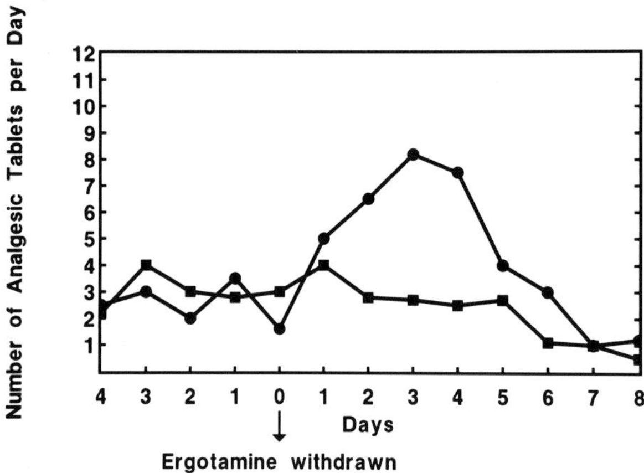

Fig. 2. Effect of concomitant naproxen; use of analgesic tablets, maximum between 2nd and 4th days of ergotamine withdrawal, effectively reduced by naproxen. *Circles*, control ($n=10$); *squares*, naproxen ($n=12$)

than Group A. However, on the 1st and 2nd nights of hospitalization, both groups showed reduced total sleep time. This is considered as an environmental factor due to the fact that they were in new surroundings in the hospital and is interpreted as "first night effect." Amounts of sedative/tranquilizers used were significantly less in Group B.

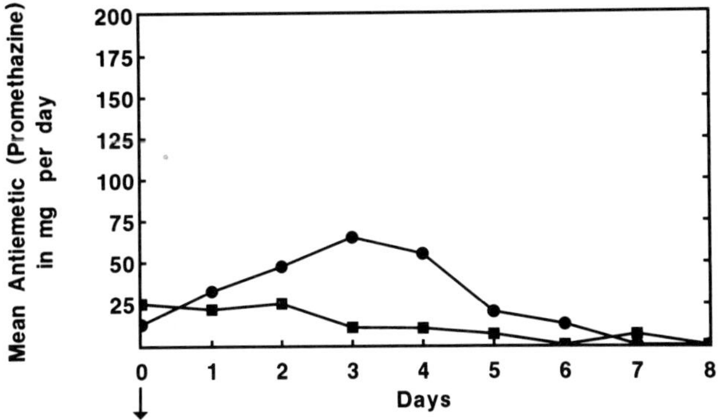

Fig. 3. Effect of concomitant naproxen – use of antiemetics. Increased antiemetic use began slightly earlier than the use of analgesics but was significantly less with the naproxen groups. *Circles*, control ($n = 10$); *squares*, naproxen ($n = 12$)

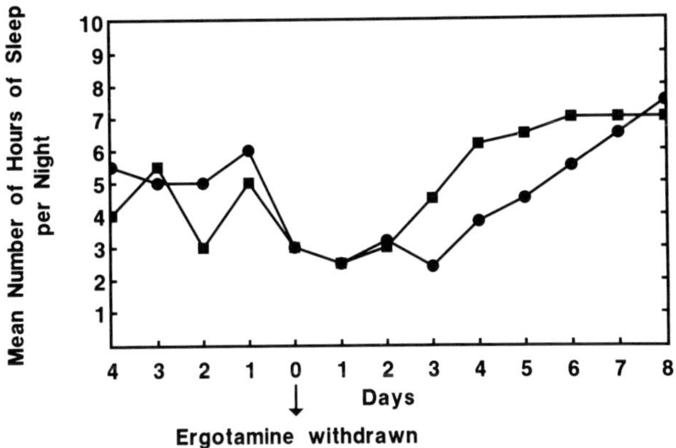

Fig. 4. Effect of concomitant naproxen; total sleep time as a measure of restlessness: note that both groups had reduced sleep on the first 2 nights in the hospital followed by better total sleep time in the naproxen groups. *Circles*, control ($n = 10$); *squares*, naproxen ($n = 12$)

Discussion

In both groups, the baseline parameters, such as the headache index, the amount of analgesics consumed, and the total sleep times, were comparable. It should be noted that both groups had daily headaches even though they were not severe. By the 8th day after withdrawal, the symptoms returned to normal in both groups, but those on naproxen had suffered less from pain, nausea, vomiting, and restlessness.

Naproxen is not tolerated well by everyone. Three patients initially included had to be dropped from the study because of the side effects. In two of them, there was severe gastric pain and aggravation of their peptic ulcers within a period of 48 h, and the third patient developed a generalized erythematous skin rash.

The mechanism of action of naproxen in the amelioration of the symptoms of ergotamine withdrawal is not clear. Welch et al. (1985) have shown that the beneficial effects of naproxen in migraine prophylaxis are probably not related to its action on platelets because the drug had no impact on platelet adhesiveness or microemboli formation, even though it effectively inhibited platelet aggregation response in most patients. They therefore postulated that the beneficial affect of naproxen in migraine may be due to a direct action on prostaglandin, blocking the vascular changes associated with migraine. Whether the prostaglandin system is directly responsible for "ergotamine headache" and symptoms of withdrawal is a matter for speculation at the present time. In any case, naproxen, a prostaglandin synthetase inhibitor, appears to be useful in the management of withdrawal symptoms.

References

Ala-Hurula V, Myllylä VV, Hokkanen E, Toloa O (1981) Tolfenamic acid and ergotamine abuse. Headache 21:240–243

Andersson P (1975) Ergotamine headache. Headache 15:118–121

Friedman AP, Brazil P, Storch TJC (1955) Ergotamine tolerance in patients with migraine. JAMA 157:881–884

Hakkarainen H, Vapaatalo H, Gothoni G, Parantainen J (1979) Tolfenamic acid is as effective as ergotamine during migraine attacks. Lancet 2:326–328

Henry P, Dartiques MP, Benetier MP, Lucas J, Duplan B, Jogeix M, Orgogozo JM (1985) Ergotamine and analgesic-induced headaches. In: Rose FC (ed) Migraine. Fifth International Migraine Symposium. Karger, Basel, pp 197–205

Hokkanen E, Waltimo O, Kallanranta T (1978) Toxic effects of ergotamine used for migraine. Headache 18:95–98

Horton BT, Peters GA (1982) Clinical manifestations of excessive use of ergotamine preparations and management of withdrawal effect. Report of 52 cases. Headache 22:214–227

Kudrow L (1982) Paradoxical effects of frequent analgesic use. Adv Neurol 33:335–341

Lippman CW (1955) Characteristic headache resulting from prolonged use of ergot derivatives. J Nerv Ment Dis 121:270–273

Mathew NT, Stubits E, Nigam MP (1982) Transformation of episodic migraine into daily headache: analysis of factors. Headache 22:66–68

Rose FC, Wilkinson M (1976) Ergotamine tartrate overdose. Br Med J [Clin Res] 1:525

Rowsell AR, Neylan C, Wilkinson M (1973) Ergotamine induced headaches in migrainous patients. Headache 13:65–67

Saper JR (1967) Migraine. II Treatment. JAMA 239:2480–2483

Tfelt-Hansen P, Krabbe AA (1981) Ergotamine abuse. Do patients benefit from withdrawal? Cephalalgia 1:29–32

Welch KM, Ellis DJ, Keenan PA (1985) Successful migraine prophylaxis with naproxen sodium. Neurology 34:1304–1310

Possible Mechanisms and Treatment
of Analgesic-Induced Chronic Headache

L. KUDROW

Introduction

Chronic muscle contraction headache is characterized by constant dull pain of at least 1 year's duration. The pain may be generalized, unilateral, vise-like, frontal or frontotemporal (Friedman et al. 1954; Lance and Curran 1964). It is often described as a nonthrobbing, pressure-type discomfort, waxing and waning throughout the day, every day, from morning until sleep. Most interesting is the frequency of analgesic use in this condition. We found that the mean daily intake of analgesic tablets consumed by 200 patients with chronic muscle contraction headaches (CMCH) was 6.2. Only 28% of patients used only simple analgesics; 38% used analgesics compounded with sedatives, tranquilizers or muscle relaxants; 31% used narcotics; and 24% used narcotic antagonists. In 36% of cases more than one type of preparation was used. Most curious was the admission of most patients that, in spite of the frequent use of analgesics, little relief was obtained (Kudrow 1982).

The effectiveness and frequency of analgesic use in an acute tension headache population (one dull headache or less per week) was compared with a subchronic tension headache group (two to four dull headaches per week) and a CMCH population (daily dull or constant dull headaches). Frequency of analgesic use was found to be proportional to frequency of headache. Effectiveness, however, was inversely proportional to frequency of analgesic use and frequency of headaches. This observation suggested that the increased use of analgesics, at some critical frequency, may contribute to the production of headache pain. The most likely mechanism for such a paradoxical effect could be explained by a negative feedback influence on the antinociceptive system, and/or by affecting cerebral biogenic amine function.

To test this hypothesis we studied 200 patients with CMCH, dividing them into two groups, amitriptyline-treated and non-treated, with two subgroups in each group, analgesic use permitted and not permitted. The rationale for evaluating the response to amitriptyline with or without analgesic use was the previously demonstrated beneficial effects of amitriptyline on CMCH (Lance et al. 1965), presumably due to its serotonergic and nonadrenergic potentiating activity, that is, the effect of amitriptyline on the cerebral biogenic amine system.

At the end of the 4-week trial, headache indices were compared between 1-month pre-trial and post-trial data for each group and subgroup. The greatest improvement (72%, $P < 0.001$) occurred in the amitriptyline-treated, nonanalgesic group, compared to a 30% improvement in the analgesic-using subgroup. Of par-

California Medical Clinic for Headache, 16542 Ventura Blvd., Encino, CA 91436, USA

Drug-Induced Headache
Ed. by H.-C. Diener and M. Wilkinson
© Springer-Verlag Berlin Heidelberg 1988

Table 1. Mean treatment responses by group and subgroup

Group	Treatment period					
	Pre-treatment HI	2nd week		4th week		Improved
		HI	HAR	HI	HAR	(%)
Amitriptyline	7.08	4.81	0.69	3.80	0.55	45[a]
+ Analgesics	6.92	5.12	0.74	4.81	0.70	30
− Analgesics	7.24	4.26	0.59	2.02	0.28	72[b]
Nonamitriptyline	7.04	5.91	0.83	5.30	0.75	25
Analgesics	7.12	6.36	0.89	5.83	0.82	18
− Analgesics	6.96	4.82	0.69	3.98	0.57	43[a]
Total						
+ Analgesics				5.33	0.76	24
− Analgesics				2.85	0.40	60[a]

HI, headache index (weekly frequency × rated intensity).
HAR, index ratio (post-treatment HI/pre-treatment HI).
[a] $P < 0.05$; [b] $P < 0.001$.

ticular note was the difference in improvement between analgesic-using and analgesic-restricted patients in the amitriptyline-withheld group. Only 18% of the former subgroup improved, compared to 43% ($P < 0.05$) of the latter group. Comparing the total analgesic-using and analgesic-restricted subgroups, a significant improvement was found for the latter only (60%, $P < 0.01$) (Table 1). Our results demonstrated that frequent analgesic use may have decreased the effectiveness of amitriptyline prophylaxis in CMCH and, indeed, may have worsened the condition in the absence of amitriptyline (Kudrow 1982).

Possible Mechanisms Explaining the Paradoxical Effect of Analgesics in CMCH

It was hypothesized that a critical frequency of analgesic use, estimated at two to three treatment days per week, may block antinociceptive activity via a negative feedback mechanisms (common to all endocrine functions), indirectly suppress biogenic amine activity and reduce the therapeutic effectiveness of amitriptyline on this system. Inherent to this hypothesis is the proposal that endogenous antinociceptive activity may include non-narcotic analgesic pathways analgous to the endorphin system, but specific to dull painful stimuli (Fig. 1). Thus, frequent use of non-narcotic analgesics may induce tachyphylaxis, tolerance and withdrawal symptoms via a negative feedback influence on a non-narcotic endogenous antinociceptive system. Finally, the results of our study and subsequent experience with a large population of patients suggests that reactivation of antinociceptive function may occur approximately 2 weeks following cessation of analgesic use, not unlike the latency period associated with return function of the thyroid gland following cessation of exogenous thyroid administration.

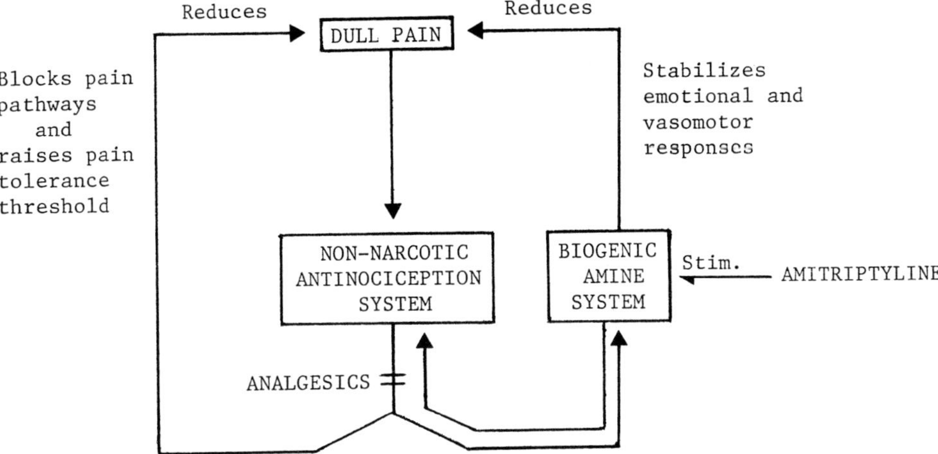

Fig. 1. Hypothetical model of paradoxical analgesic-induced chronic headache. It is postulated that under normal conditions dull pain should stimulate non-narcotic antinociceptive activity directly to affect inhibition of pain conduction, and indirectly to stabilize emotional and vasomotor responses via biogenic amine activity. It is further hypothesized that exogenous analgesics, used at a critical frequency, may inhibit, by negative feedback, antinociceptive activity and consequently biogenic amine stimulation. The consequence of critically frequent analgesic use may present the clinical picture of chronic muscle contraction headaches: persistent dull headaches, emotional instability, and vasomotor lability. Discontinuance of analgesics may suffice to reverse this condition, but may require potentiation of concomitant treatment with low doses of amitriptyline

In a more recent survey (Kudrow and Esperanca 1987, unpublished) we demonstrated that continued restriction of analgesics and amitriptyline maintenance provided continued relief from headaches. Indeed, discontinuance of amitriptyline (after a minimum of 3 months on medications) often resulted in continued relief.

The rapid response to analgesic restriction and low-dose amitriptyline therapy and continued relief following cessation of amitriptyline suggests that factors which initiate the muscle contraction headache condition may not be responsible for chronicity. It is possible that in an earlier period, extrinsic/intrinsic physical or psychopersonality factors (trauma, crises, surgery, illness, or chronic stress) may have precipitated the disorder, but these were no longer the driving force. It is our contention that suppression of antinociception and biogenic amine function due to a critical frequency of analgesic use was responsible for increasing and sustaining chronic headache pain.

Treatment

Management of analgesic-induced chronic headaches includes: (a) discontinuance of analgesics; (b) low-dose amitriptyline medication; (c) record keeping; and (d) follow-up visits. Perhaps it is most important, however, to offer the patients a scientific model to explain the pathogenesis of their disorder, the deleterious effects of analgesics and the neuropharmacology of amitriptyline. At our clinic this is provided in great detail.

Amitriptyline. Amitriptyline is prescribed in a subantidepressant dosage. It is reportedly more efficacious in lower doses (10–25 mg) than in antidepressant doses (50–100 mg) (Holland et al. 1983). The reason for this phenomenon is unknown. We have speculated, however, that the ratio of serotonergic to noradrenergic receptor blockade may be dose dependent.

Subantidepressant doses of amitriptyline are prescribed in a nightly dose of 10–20 mg. Even at this low dose, patients are aware of the three major side effects: mouth dryness, sluggishness upon awakening, and weight gain, secondary to an increased appetite.

Discontinuance of Analgesics. Analgesics are discontinued abruptly since tapering of medication is usually associated with a greater frequency of recidivism. Amitriptyline is started simultaneously. An increase in headaches should be expected the 1st week following withdrawal, which may also be attended by vasomotor symptoms and emotional changes. A significant reduction in headaches and other symptoms should occur by the 2nd week. A marked improvement over pretreatment status should be observed after the 2nd week.

Record Keeping. It is imperative that patients maintain a daily diary of headache attacks since it provides the most objective record of improvement for both the patient and clinician. Notation of menstrual days on the headache diary aids in the recognition of associated hormonal migraine attacks. These are apt to occur from 3 days premenstrually to as late as 2 days after the last menstrual day. Hormonal migraine may also occur a day following ovulation.

Follow-Up Visits. At our clinic, patients are seen in follow-up 1 month after the initial visit. Subsequent revisits occur at increasing intervals depending on the rate of improvement. As determined by the headache diary, if the patient has achieved a low sustained headache frequency, the amitriptyline medication is tapered and ultimately discontinued.

Experience has shown that in patients who improve significantly, becoming stationary after 6 months, the stationary state can be maintained without amitriptyline medication in the majority of cases. Some patients will relapse within the following 2 years, but almost never to the pre-treatment headache frequency rate. Of a total population of patients thus treated, approximately 50% continue to be relatively headache free following discontinuation of medication and they are discharged from our clinic.

Summary

Evidence for a relationship between frequent non-narcotic analgesic use and headache chronicity was presented. A hypothesis was suggested to explain the mechanisms of this phenomenon. It was postulated that a critical rate of analgesic use may inhibit central nonendorphin antinociceptive and biogenic amine activity. A successful treatment regimen for analgesic-induced chronic headaches was described. It includes discontinuance of analgesics and low-dose amitriptyline medication.

References

Friedman AP, von Storch TUC, Merritt HH (1954) Migraine and tension headaches. A clinical study of two thousand cases. Neurology 4:773–788
Holland JV, Holland CV, Kudrow L (1983) Low-dose amitriptyline prophylaxis in chronic scalp muscle contraction headache. Proc 1st International Headache Congress, Munich, p 134
Kudrow L (1982) Paradoxical effects of frequent analgesic use. In: Critchley M, Friedman A, Gorini S, Sicuteri F (eds) Advances in neurology, vol 33. Raven, New York, pp 335–451
Lance JW, Curran DA (1964) Treatment of chronic tension headache. Lancet 1:1236–1239
Lance JW, Curran DA, Anthony M (1965) Investigations into the mechanism and treatment of chronic headache. Med J Aust 2:909–916

Characteristics and Treatment
of Analgesic Rebound Headache

A. M. Rapoport and R. E. Weeks

The frequent and excessive use of non-narcotic analgesics such as aspirin and acetaminophen in chronic headache sufferers often perpetuates and worsens head pain rather than relieving it. It also interferes with standard, usually effective, pharmacologic therapy and prevents expected improvement. While small amounts of analgesics may initially offer some relief in scalp muscle contraction headache, individuals with frequent pain seem to habituate to the therapeutic actions of such agents. This begins a cycle of increased intake to achieve similar relief.

At some point, increased consumption not only fails to provide pain reduction, but it begins to perpetuate and intensify headaches. This paradoxical effect of analgesics is called "analgesic rebound headache." The term "rebound" refers both to the worsening of the headache in 3–4 h as the apparent analgesic effect of the medication wears off, and to the fact that the patient goes through a marked exacerbation (almost a withdrawal phenomenon) after medication is stopped totally. This worsening usually continues for 5–14 days or more, which is the average length of the analgesic washout period before the patient begins to improve.

Most patients with analgesic rebound headaches are in their 30s or 40s and have a history of mild chronic scalp muscle contraction headache prior to abusing analgesics. Many also have a history of intermittent migraine. They usually experience two to four mild headaches per week in addition to their occasional migraine attacks. These headaches last from 6 h to all day and are described as a mild, dull, bilateral, frontal-occipital, or diffuse discomfort. They are not associated with visual complaints or autonomic symptoms such as nausea, vomiting, diarrhea, sweating, pupillary changes, or stuffed nostrils. There is usually a steady, nonthrobbing pain, and there are no focal symptoms such as weakness, paresthesias, or speech problems.

These patients gradually begin to use over-the-counter or prescription analgesics in larger amounts. They note only temporary and partial relief and begin to medicate three or four times per day as relief wears off quickly. Some start to take medication in anticipation of a severe headache so that they can function. After several months, their mild scalp muscle contraction headache becomes moderately severe. The patient awakens with it and goes to bed with it, but it waxes and wanes throughout the day. It, too, is not associated with nausea, vomiting, or other migraine symptoms. Occasionally, it is severe and throbbing.

Analgesics, which were taken two times per day in small quantities with relief early in the course of the headache, are now taken regularly, habitually, and in

The New England Center for Headache, 40 East Putnam Avenue, Cos Cob, CT 06807, USA

Drug-Induced Headache
Ed. by H.-C. Diener and M. Wilkinson
© Springer-Verlag Berlin Heidelberg 1988

excessive amounts. Patients frequently awaken in the morning with a headache and medicate before getting out of bed. They continue to medicate every 3–4 h until bedtime. They may take a handful of pills at once. There is little relief, and the headache appears to worsen in spite of increased amounts of medication. It is curious that patients continue to take in large amounts, medications which do not appear to help them. Many report a partial, temporary reduction in their pain level for 1–4 h after taking analgesics. Most patients admit that this is a habit that they have gotten into, and which is difficult to break.

Original Studies

Kudrow (1982) first addressed the paradoxical effect of frequent analgesic use. He studied the effect of stopping analgesics in daily headache sufferers, both in patients placed on amitriptyline and those not. He studied 200 patients with chronic scalp muscle contraction headache. The first group of 100 received amitriptyline and the second group of 100 did not. At the end of 4 weeks, the amitriptyline-treated group had a mean improvement of 30% in the analgesic-using group in contrast to 72% in the analgesic-restricted group. In the nonamitriptyline-treated group, the corresponding figures were 18% and 43%. These results indicated that it is essential to take patients off their analgesics even when they are appropriately treated with amitriptyline.

New England Center for Headache Clinical Studies

In our first clinical study on analgesic rebound headache, we randomly selected 20 patients with analgesic rebound headache who completed at least 4 months of therapy while keeping daily headache index calendars. For this review, we defined "analgesic rebound headache" as a daily headache in patients who used a minimum of 20 analgesic tablets per week (most usually either aspirin, acetaminophen or Fiorinal) and, rarely, narcotics.

At the end of the study, the patients were divided into three groups. The pure analgesic rebound group was made up of those who experienced at least a 50% decrease in daily, mild to moderate headaches over the 4-month period of observation simply by discontinuing their analgesics. The chronic scalp muscle contraction/depressive group experienced at least a 50% reduction in daily, mild to moderate headaches, but only after discontinuing analgesics *and* being placed on a tricyclic antidepressant, either amitriptyline or doxepin. The treatment failure group continued to have daily, mild to moderate headaches despite discontinuing the analgesics and being given trials of an antidepressant. None of these patients were given biofeedback training during the 4 months of data collection.

At the end of the 4th month, the pure rebound headache patients continued to improve on no medication. The chronic scalp muscle contraction headache patients improved further and were still on their tricyclic antidepressants, and the treatment failure group was no better.

A study was made of the Minnesota Multiphasic Personality Inventory (MMPI) of these patients. The pure rebound headache patients tended to be hypochondriacal and were probably healthy and nervous about their symptoms. The scalp muscle contraction headache/depressive headache patients had many symptoms but appeared not to be concerned about them or denied them. They probably had a masked depression and were unaware of it. The high K scale, which is a validity scale, indicated that they are rather defensive individuals. The treatment failure group included individuals who were hysterical and histrionic. They talked about their pain, had low energy levels, and did not seem to be depressed. Their pain seemed to come from other sources, possibly secondary gain, or other problems in their life.

In a second study at The New England Center for Headache, we reviewed 70 analgesic rebound headache patients whom we defined as patients with daily headaches who were taking 14 or more analgesic tablets per week. We tracked their headache indices over a 4-month period after they discontinued all analgesics. Some were not given any other treatment and were simply observed. Some were treated with 2 mg cyproheptadine (Periactin) and 50 mg vitamin B_6. Some were treated with 10–30 mg amitriptyline (Elavil) at night. The composition of the group was 56 females and 14 males. Their average age was 39.5 years, and the average age of onset of headache was 25.8 years. The average duration of headache was 13 years. These patients took an average of 36 analgesic tablets per week and their caffeine intake was over 800 mg per day. In this study, we defined a "significant decrease" in headache as a 67% reduction in the frequency of daily, mild to moderate headache. At the end of 1 month, the results indicated improvement in four patients who were taking no medication, 24 patients on cyproheptadine and vitamine B_6, and 18 patients on amitriptyline. In all, 46 of 70 patients improved at the end of 1 month. This is 65.7% of the sample number. Their baseline frontal EMG levels were not significantly different using a *t* test.

At the end of the 2nd month, three more patients on Periactin and vitamin B_6 had significant improvement and eight more patients on amitriptyline improved. Thus, 11 more patients in the sample improved during the 2nd month. In total, there were 57 of 70 (81.4% of the sample) patients who had improved significantly at the end of 2nd months. Although we knew from our previous work that one-third of analgesic rebound headache patients would improve simply by stopping their pain medication, we felt it necessary to treat some of these patients with amitriptyline, Periactin, or vitamin B_6 to make their withdrawal less uncomfortable. Although giving these medications decreases the purity of the groups, we do feel it is appropriate to medicate patients for their comfort.

Analgesic Washout Period

No study to date has examined the length of time that the analgesic detoxification may take following cessation of pain medication. Such data are important as the presence of analgesics appears to compromise otherwise effective headache treatment and, therefore, may cause a delay in symptom reduction due to the detoxification process. Such information is vital in terms of awareness of what an adequate length of treatment trial is before a drug regimen should be considered "ineffective."

The third clinical study at The New England Center for Headache addressed this situation. Ninety patients took part in our study of the analgesic washout period. The group was composed of 69 females and 21 males which is a typical sample of the patients that we treat at our Center. All patients fit our criteria for analgesic rebound headache which were: (a) almost constant, daily, mild to severe, generalized headache; and (b) patients taking more than 14 analgesic tablets per week. These patients averaged 35 analgesic tablets per week, and a typical patient had experienced this type of headache for an average of 9 years. Their average age was 39. Again, we defined "significant improvement" as greater than a 67% reduction in the frequency of daily head pain. By definition, the patients started out with approximately 30 days of head pain per month and they would, therefore, have to have fewer than 10 headache days per month to reach this criterion of significant improvement.

A substantial number of patients improved by merely discontinuing their analgesics. Some improved rapidly in the 1st month while others did not reach the criterion until week 12. Depending on the clinical picture, some patients were again treated with cyproheptadine and vitamin B_6 while others were given small doses of amitriptyline (10–30 mg at hour of sleep).

Physiological readings from the four subgroups showed no significant differences between their baseline EMG readings of the frontalis muscles with eyes open and eyes closed. The nonimproved group showed a slightly higher EMG level. Finger temperature as an index of peripheral blood flow yielded no significant differences. MMPI testing of the 90 patients representing their personality profiles showed no statistical difference between groups. However, an interesting trend emerged with the nonimproved group which showed almost significant elevations of scales 1, 2, and 3, indicative of a chronic pain profile. This is a trend that will have to be investigated further. We are not able to predict subgroup membership on the basis of either the physiological or psychological data.

Results show that there were impressive improvement rates consistently through months 1, 2, and 3, independent of medication (cyproheptadine, amitriptyline, and vitamin B_6) or no medication. A total of 82% of patients improved. The data suggest that the analgesic washout period may take as long as 12 weeks. It is our conclusion that, to fully evaluate any headache treatment modality, a trial of 12 weeks utilizing that modality, after cessation of analgesic medication, is necessary when treating patients who have analgesic rebound headache as part of their clinical picture. Also, when doing research studies, one should not use the number of analgesic tablets as a treatment outcome issue.

Discussion

The pain of chronic scalp muscle contraction headache was thought at one time to be peripheral in nature, coming from contracted muscles and painful nerves in the head and neck (Simons et al. 1943). Many now feel that it may be a central nervous system disorder. The analgesics may be more centrally active than the peripheral role they play in inhibiting prostaglandins. In fact, aspirin and acetaminophen do work centrally to relieve pain and lower body temperature. Toxic doses do cause central side effects.

Our own studies have shown that some patients with chronic scalp muscle contraction headaches have high levels of muscle contraction, but some have very low levels. A significant subgroup of these patients tend to be depressed. Scalp muscle contraction headache may, therefore, be several different entities, only some of which are related to scalp muscles and some to brain mechanisms.

If we consider the pain of chronic scalp muscle contraction headache to be central in origin and we accept the concept that excessive use of non-narcotic analgesics is associated with tolerance, habituation, and rebound pain, then we can postulate that the pain is secondary to suppression of a central antinociceptive system. The most likely system affected is the serotonergic system controlling sleep, dull pain, and feeling of well-being, as suggested by Sicuteri (Sicuteri 1972; Sicuteri et al. 1973). This system may be analogous to the endorphin system which controls more severe pain (Hole and Berge 1981). Amitriptyline affects this system by preventing the reuptake of serotonin into nerve terminals and thereby increasing its concentration and prolonging its effects (Diamond and Baltes 1971). It is known that aspirin increases central serotonin levels. It used to be thought that the rate-limiting step in the availability of cerebral serotonin was the conversion of the amino acid tryptophan to serotonin by the enzyme 5-tryptophan hydroxylase. It is now known that the availability of tryptophan in the brain is the limiting factor of the level of cerebral serotonin.

Tryptophan is the only amino acid circulating in plasma which is highly bound to serum proteins. Salicylates (aspirin) break that bond and increase the availability of free tryptophan. Studies show that 1–2 h after administration of tryptophan there is an increase in brain serotonin (Tagliamonte 1973; Tagliamonte et al. 1973). But there is a paradoxical effect with increased pain. The mechanism is not well understood. Possibly, there is a down-regulation of serotonin receptor sites with a reduction in the number of such sites in the brain, thereby reducing the effectiveness of the increased amount of serotonin.

It is possible that pharmacologic conditioning and learning play an important part in understanding the analgesic rebound phenomenon. About 4 h after taking medication, the patient may unconsciously feel the need to have more medication and may, therefore, feel pain until this medication is taken.

Implications for Therapy

It is extremely important to take an accurate history of medication intake. Most patients will not tell their physician that they are taking aspirin, acetaminophen, or other over-the-counter analgesics unless specifically asked. Sometimes they do not even consider these drugs as medications. When asked, they will usually minimize the true quantity that they are taking. If the physician is not aware that the patient is taking analgesics, his treatment will not take into account the syndrome of analgesic rebound headache and, therefore, may be totally ineffective. Once it is documented that the patients are taking large amounts of analgesics, it is essential that they be withdrawn from these medications completely. Although they can be taken off their analgesics abruptly, providing they are not taking narcotics, it has been our habit to taper them gradually over a 3–5-day period. We tend to substitute vasoactive medications and mild sedatives which may be only acting as placebo, but do appear to help the patient.

These patients must be carefully educated on more than one occasion and they must understand that they will probably worsen for several days before they begin to improve. It is also important to follow up with these patients in approximately 2–4 weeks to make sure that they are keeping themselves off the analgesics. Many of them do not and will relapse at some point in time.

The analgesic rebound phenomenon is very interesting and rather pervasive. It seems to occur in most civilized countries in the world, and only the names and the composition of the medication seem to change from country to country. The headache specialist who makes use of his knowledge of analgesic rebound headache to help his patients is often much more effective then the one who does not.

References

Diamond S, Baltes BJ (1971) Chronic tension headache treated with amitriptyline – a double blind study. Headache 11:110–116

Hole K, Berge O (1981) Regulation of pain sensitivity in the central nervous system. Cephalalgia 1:51–59

Kudrow L (1982) Paradoxical effects of frequent analgesic use. In: Critchley M (ed) Advances in neurology, vol 33. Raven, New York, pp 335–341

Sicuteri F (1972) Headache as possible expression of deficiency of brain 5-hydroxy-tryptamine (central denervation supersensitivity). Headache 12:69–72

Sicuteri F, Anselmi B, Del Bianco PL (1973) 5-Hydroxytryptamine supersensitivity as a new theory of headache and central pain: a clinical pharmacological approach with p-chlorophenylalanine. Psychopharmacology (Berlin) 29:347

Simons DJ, Day E, Goodell H, Wolff HG (1943) Experimental studies on headache: muscles of the scalp and neck as sources of pain. Assoc Res Nerv Dis Proc 23:228–244

Tagliamonte A (1973) Increase in brain tryptophan and stimulation of serotonin synthesis by salicylate. J Neurochem 20:909–912

Tagliamonte A, Biggio G, Vargiu, Gessa GL (1973) Free tryptophan in serum controls, brain tryptophan level and serotonin synthesis. Life Sci 12:277–287

Conclusions

M. WILKINSON

The problems of headache due to drug abuse have been discussed in this book. Now that the problem has been delineated, efforts must be made to deal with it. As with all drug dependencies the best treatment is to discontinue the drug immediately and dissuade the patient from taking it again in the future. Admitting the patient to hospital for a period of 7–14 days is usually sufficient to deal with the immediate problems, but long-term care is necessary in the majority of cases if the patient is not to return to taking the same drugs. The substitution of different types of medication has been used, and in the case of analgesic abuse good results have been reported from the use of beta-blockers, calcium channel blockers and antidepressants. Where the patient is depressed, amitriptyline is probably the drug of choice.

In all headache patients an accurate diagnosis must be made as, in my opinion, the treatment of migraine, either classical or common, is different from that of tension or muscle contraction headache. In the majority of patients suffering from migraine, therapy for the acute attack is all that is necessary as it is very unusual for patients to have more than six attacks of migraine a month. For these patients, treatment of the attack is rest, metoclopramide or domperidone and either aspirin or paracetamol. In about 30% of sufferers 1 or 2 mg ergotamine, given as a suppository or by inhalation, may also be required. Ergotamine should not be used on more than two occasions in any 1 week. The patients with a combination of migraine and tension headache or those with tension headache or muscle contraction headache are much more difficult to treat. Ergot and its derivatives should only be given to patients with migraine as these drugs are effective only for migraine. Patients should be warned against the frequent use of analgesics.

If migraine attacks occur more than twice a month, prophylactic therapy may be indicated, and there is now a variety of drugs which may be used. These include the beta-blockers (propranolol, metoprolol), the calcium channel blockers (e.g. nimodipine and flunarizine) and pizotifen. Good results have been obtained from all of these. Persistent daily headache may be a symptom of depression, and for these patients an anti-depressant may be used. Also, some patients are helped by relaxation techniques such as meditation or biofeedback, and also by acupuncture. The advantage of these treatments is that they do not lead to chronic drug abuse.

One interesting aspect of this problem is the difference in drug usage in different countries. In the United Kingdom, partly due to government regulations,

The City of London Migraine Clinic, 22 Charterhouse Square, London, ECIM 6DX, United Kingdom

Drug-Induced Headache
Ed. by H.-C. Diener and M. Wilkinson
© Springer-Verlag Berlin Heidelberg 1988

there are relatively few compound preparations, i.e. those containing a mixture of analgesics, barbiturates and caffeine, and possibly as a result of this, chronic drug abuse for headache is not as great a problem as it is elsewhere. The advice given to medical practitioners in the United Kingdom is that the use of barbiturates or diazepines should be avoided where possible because dependence and tolerance can readily occur. Many headache preparations which contain barbiturates are freely available in other countries, and two of the most popular are Optalidon and Fiorinal. Phenazone is another drug which has been banned in some countries, but not in others. If the use of these drugs can be limited, one cause of drug abuse headache can be eliminated.

Subject Index